Chakras For Beginners

The Complete Beginner's Guide for Understanding and Balance the 7 Chakras. Exercises For Opening Your Chakras Quickly and Easily. How to Use Chakra Stones on Yourself

Introduction

Congratulations on purchashing Chakra For Beginners

I am pleased that you have chosen the popular chakra technique to enable you to live in peace and harmony with yourself and other people. Chakras are basically the "spinning wheels of energy" which create the combination of life force and energy. There are many chakras in our body, but only seven chakras are well-known and popularly discussed. They include the root, sacral, solar plexus, the heart, the throat, the third eye, and the crown head chakras.

When all the chakras are balanced and spinning smoothly, a person experiences a wonderful life mentally, physically, emotionally. The body, mind, and soul are all functioning well. A person with a balanced chakra will have excellent relationships, goals, interests, and conversations flowing with ease.

On the other hand, when our chakras are misaligned or imbalanced, we become over-active or under-active, and life will have a lot of challenges. The misaligned chakra will not easily show, and you might not see it on the surface. However, if you take time to practice, learn, or visit a professional healer, you will be able to recognize your problematic chakra.

There are different remedies that are known and available to any individual who wishes to align or balance the misaligned chakras. Some of them include yoga, meditation, exercises, and even the foods and diet we consume.

The seven chakras are parts that we cannot see, but we can feel and touch them. These are parts that help us get intuition, create our being, help us deal with our relationships and among other things as discussed.

The chakra topic is wide and in-depth. All seven chakras also have different colors that correspond to each one of them.

The chakras enable us to fully understand ourselves. Scientific studies are also linking some of the previous untested human attributes that have been practiced in chakra for centuries.

Chapter 1: What Are Chakras?

Chakra is a Sanskrit (one of India's 22 official languages and Hinduism's liturgical semantic) word which literally means the "wheel" or "disk." In yoga, meditation, and Reiki practices, chakras which originated in India as far as between 1500 and 500 BC, are referenced to as the spiritual energy centers within the body of a human being. There are seven main energy centers or chakras in the body aligning from the spine; they start at the bottom of the spine through to the body, neck, and to the crown or the top of the head.

Each of the seven chakras corresponds to particular organs in providing the right energy as well as to your spiritual, emotional, physical, and psychological states of life. The chakras influence and empower all parts of your life. Within the chakras, there is "prana," which is the vital force of life and the ultimate healing energy which is within us and around us to keep us vibrant, healthy, alive and happy. The seven chakras are swirling wheels of energy, and if there is a blockage, the flow of energy or "prana" stops, and it can lead to illness.

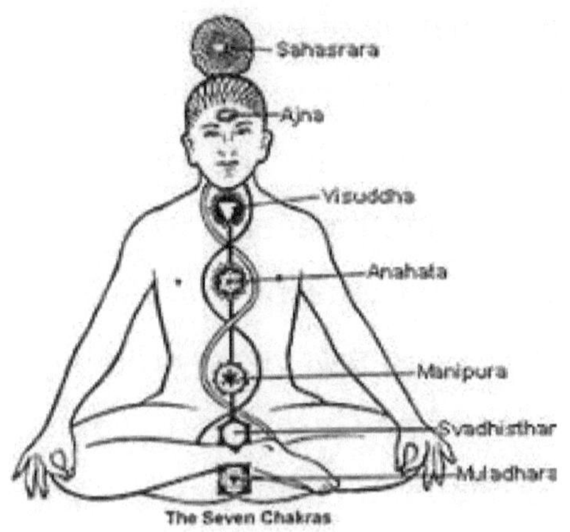

What Are The Seven Chakras?

Leaning the seven chakras will help you tune with the natural and spiritual energy cycles of your body. Having knowledge will also enable you to balance the chakras and live a harmonious and healthy life. When learning and exploring the chakras, you should start from the beginning. We are going to start from the first chakra, which is the base of the spine all the way up to the crown of the head.

The 1st Chakra-Root Chakra-Muladhara

Muladhara is the combination of two Sanskrit words, which is "Mula" and "Dhara" which means the roots and support respectively. The role of the root chakra is to connect human energy with the Earth, which is also known as the foundational base or grounding. The 1st root or chakra root is located at the base of the spine just close to your tailbone or coccygeal region. It encompasses the first three vertebrae and the pelvic floor. Root chakra will give you boldness and courage to tackle new challenges with ease.

In our modern world today, the first chakra will give you everything you need as a human being to survive and pursue new ventures or major life goals. In our modern world, it also translates to emotional and financial security in many ways. In other terms, when your root chakra is balanced, you will have a balanced feeling and feel a sense of peace and accomplishment when you think about things like shelter, safety, and money. Our relationship with Mother Nature is defined in this root, and Earth is its element. It is associated with the color red.

In some cases, the root chakra can get blocked, and this will cause a feeling of threat, anxiousness, and panic. The anxiety will infiltrate through your mind, and a feeling of uncertainty is created. You will not succeed in putting all your focus on one particular thing because of constant worries about your well-being. To some people, it might appear as general paranoia or hypochondria. It might also cause physical issues like low energy levels, sore lower back, cold extremities, digestive problems, and hip pain. When the first chakra is open, you will feel safe.

The 2nd Chakra-Sacral Chakra-Svadhishana

Sacral chakra translates to "the place of the self" and is the second in the order. It is located below the navel and just above the pubic bone. It is all about human identity and creativity. It is here in the second chakra that the force to enrich yourself through creativity and to enjoy life stems from in our lives. Sacra chakra is associated with water as it's element.

When Sacral Chakra is in balance, you will abundantly enjoy and nurture practices of pleasurable aspects of your life existence such as intimacy and sex and other things like good food without overdoing them. You will get a feeling of fulfillment, pleasure, happiness, wellness, joy, and abundance for pursuing creativity and pleasurable things. The second chakra is associated with an orange color and is depicted as a lotus, which is orange in color and has six petals. Sacral chakra as a form of energetic function also helps us regulate our desires and emotions.

Sacral Chakra might also get blocked or misaligned, and it might happen if you are experiencing some form of emotional stability, restlessness, boredom, or feeling of lack of inspiration to get creative. It can also misalign as a result of an unsatisfying relationship, any form of sexuality stress like low sex drive or sexual dysfunction, fear of change, addiction-like behavior, hormonal imbalance, obesity, gambling-problem, and increased allergies.

The 3rd Chakra-Solar Plexus-Manipura

Its Manipura name is Sanskrit word, which means "lustrous gem." It is a source of personal power, self-confidence, self-esteem, and self-worth. Solar Plexus or Manipura is located in the upper part of the abdomen from the belly button to the base of the chest just at a point where your two sets of ribs connect. It is associated with yellow. The Solar Plexus is also the source of the person's sense of true identity. It is also associated with the element of fire and it as connection with energy as well.

When Solar Plexus is balanced, you will feel powerful and have a feeling of a great sense of wisdom. It is said to have a direct influence on our professional and personal success. The energetic function is to optimize human power so that we can steer our lives with determination, confidence, and strength. Solar Plexus chakra enables us to control our lives. The third chakra is also responsible for all things related to our stomach, including digesting our food, metabolic process, and any other stomach-related issue. It enables us to digest our experiences the same way it does to the food we consume, helping us overcome the challenges, utilize any opportunities, and make informed and wise decisions.

Your third chakra might get blocked or overactive, and when this happens, you will have low self-esteem, have control or anger issues, lack of empathy or compassion or feel too energized as well. You will also tend to feel bad about yourself, and someone can take advantage of you easily. Physically, you will encounter digestive issues such as stomachaches or gas problems. You might also experience imbalances in your organs like liver, kidneys, and pancreas.

The 4th Chakra-Heart-Anahata

Anahata is a Sanskrit word meaning "unstruck" or "unhurt." It is located directly over the human heart, down your breastbone and then goes up to the throat. It is said to exist at the center of your chest. It is in the middle of all the seven chakras connecting the lower chakras (physical world) and the higher chakras (the heaven). The fourth chakra represents where the spiritual and physical meet. It is associated with color green and air as its element. The fourth or heart chakra is the source of love, kindness, and compassion. It is also a source of connection, and it's where we get influences for our personal and professional relationships. The Heart Chakra is also associated with openness, joy, and peace.

It also serves as the bridge between our mind, emotions, body, and spirit. The fourth chakra is connected to several other glands including thymus and lymph glands.

When your heart chakra is balanced and aligned, love, and compassion for yourself and others flow freely. You will still continue to show kindness and compassion to others, even when things are tough or go against your wish.

When the heart chakra is blocked, you find yourself giving way to anger, hatred, jealousy, fear of betrayal or distrust and other negative emotions towards yourself and others. Holding a grudge against yourself or others is also a sign of misaligned or blocked Heart chakra. The blockage of the fourth heart is the reason why relationships are ruined and why people harbor negative feelings. The physical symptoms associated with misaligned Heart Chakra include heartburn, fast heart rate, palpitations, and interpersonal confrontations and issues.

The 5th Chakra-Throat-Vishuddha

Vishuddha is a Sanskrit word which means "very or especially pure." It is located in the throat area. The fifth chakra is also associated with the neck, mouth, jaw, parathyroid, thyroid, larynx, and tongue. The Throat Chakra is all about speaking and expressing your inner truth. It ensures you are able to express your voice of truth and feelings with confidence and that you are able to communicate with others appropriately. It is associated with the color blue, and it's also connected with our ability to listen as we communicate and to empathize.

When your Throat Chakra is balanced, you will express yourself with a clear voice, confidence, truth, kindness, and love. You will also listen to others attentively; use kind and appropriate words when responding. The Fifth Chakra enables you to speak with wisdom and share with those around you to inspire and enlighten them.

When the Throat Chakra is blocked, you will not pay attention or stay focused in your communications; you will have a problem expressing yourself and speaking the truth. You will find it hard to share your thoughts, or you might feel those around you are ignoring what you are saying. Physically, you will find yourself raising your voice unnecessarily; you may also suffer sore throat or throat infections, thyroid issues, mouth ulcers, tension headaches, or shoulder or neck stiffness.

The 6th Chakra-The Third Eye-Ajna

Ajna is a Sanskrit word which means "beyond wisdom." The Third Eye or the Sixth Chakra is responsible for opening up our minds for more information beyond our five senses and the material world. The Third-Eye is the center and the governor of our intuition. The chakra gives us our capacity to identify and tap into it. This chakra is located between your eyes. The Third Eye is also accountable for several organ functionalities, which include head, eyes, pituitary gland, head and lower part of the brain. The pituitary gland is a small pine cone-shaped gland in a human brain and is responsible for taking in light and assisting you to stay awake during the day and sleepy at night.

Ajna Chakra is symbolized by the color indigo and often associated with the human ability to use logic, rationalize, utilize a sense of thought and reach a reasonable conclusion after wise analysis. When your Third Eye Chakra is balanced, you will have a clear picture and feel in tune with your energetic and physical world.

When your Third Eye Chakra is blocked, you will find it hard to access your intuition, recalling vital facts, have trust issues with your inner voice, and have difficulty in learning new techniques. It is also the bridge between you and the world outside or beyond us, and it enables us to cut through dramas and illusions to get a clear picture. One thing that makes your Third Eye Chakra unique unlike other chakras is that when other lower chakras (from the 1st to 5th chakras) are unbalanced, your Third Eye may equally get unbalanced as well.

Unbalanced Sixth Chakra might also cause you to act introverted, more judgmental, anxious, depressed, and dismissive. Physically, you might experience dizziness, headaches, or any other brain-related health issue.

The 7th Chakra-Crown-Sahasrara

Sahasrara translates to "thousand pelated." It connects our consciousness with that of the rest of the world. It is located at the very top of the crown of your head. It is associated with the light element, and it's the center of our enlightenment and spiritual linking to the divine, others, and our higher selves. It is often very hard to understand this Seventh Chakra, but you can think of it as magnetism. The consciousness of our universe is pulled by an energetic pull to our human consciousness. It is associated with a violet color.

When the Crown Chakra is balanced, any realizations which you will experience will happen along the lines of consciousness, awareness, all expansive and undivided. It also provides humans with some very powerful potentials and abilities. It is open to unlimited power, and it is believed the people are at different levels of attaining their total enlightenment, but all of us are in the same journey.

Focusing on other chakras will greatly help in aligning all components of your spiritual, emotional, and physical existence. This is advisable if you wish to move several steps further and faster in getting the ultimate enlightenment rather than trying to seek universal consciousness directly. Put all your focus on balancing other chakras to achieve balancing your Crown Chakra and achieve greater ultimate enlightenment.

When your Seventh Chakra is cannot get overactive, but when blocked, you will have a feeling of emotional distress and isolation. You can also feel well and okay, even when your Crown Chakra is not fully balanced, which is also very normal.

Using Meditation to Help Your Chakras

Chakras are the bridge between physical manifestation of invisible energy and the mind-body connection. Tuning in to our body's different areas will satisfy chakras' needs to get them into balance, and there are several ways to harness meditation power to achieve this goal.

Meditation for Root Chakra

Practicing meditation tactics that will connect to the Earth is what will help you get your chakra into balance. Your meditation practices should focus on the energy on your feet that will balance your body and anchor you to safety.

One of the meditation practices is to stand up and straighten your body, adjust your feet and shoulder width apart as you slightly bend your knees. Retain your body balance and move your pelvis forward just a bit to evenly distribute your weight over your feet's soul. Direct your weight forward and remain in this position for several minutes. Relax and chant the word "LAM." Hold breath and release, and at the end of the meditation, you should feel confident and ready to pursue your life goals.

Mediation for Sacral Chakra

The mediation technique for Sacral Chakra involves visualizing as if you are pulling the cords out of your body from the location of this chakra in your body, which is below the navel area. Sage your space after cutting the cords and visualize holding a carnelian crystal in your hands, take three deep breaths as your eyes remain closed. Say in silent your head or aloud "I request the highest vibration of light and love to connect with my highest clear self and clear all unwanted energy and I command the crystal to balance my Sacral Chakra." You will have pictures in your mind of color orange filling up in your second chakra space while healing with balanced light.

Meditation for Solar Plexus Chakra

Your meditation techniques should focus on helping you with your confidence. Solar Plexus Chakra meditation is best done in the morning. Start by deep-belly breathing while seated. Visualize your day ahead as you meditate using deep breath and tuned body. Visualize the things you need to do in your day and other important things you need to take care of in the coming days. If it's sunny, perform this form of Solar Plexus for the light to fill in your body and enable the sunrays to shine on your chakra as you think about how to succeed in your undertakings.

Meditation for Heart Chakra

There are different meditation practices that you can perform for the Heart Chakra. Sit on your knees quietly and put your hands directly at the center of your chest. Silently chant the sound "YAM" while thinking about the fourth or the Heart Chakra and what it stands for, which is love. Continue performing this meditation practice until you feel relaxed and you feel "clean" again and ready to show love and compassion.

Meditation for Throat Chakra

You will need the use of crystals when meditating for chakra. You are required to hold blue calcite or turquoise or lace agate with your left hand, which will receive the crystal's energy during meditation. You will have to sit on your knees as you meditate and focus on the position of the Throat Chakra which is at the base of your throat. You can also meditate and concentrate on your throat while placing your crystal on chakra's position. You can also use essential oils that are said to honor Throat Chakra, and they include rosemary, lavender, German Chamomile, hyssop, and Frankincense.

Mediation for Third-Eye Chakra

Sit up and straighten your spine while in a comfortable position and cross your legs. You can either sit in a chair or on the floor. Rest your hands on your knees and make sure your chest is wide open. Rest your tongue on the mouth floor behind your front teeth. Your index finger should also touch your thumb and then breathe deeply, slowly and smoothly. Put all your focus to the Third Eye and even when other thoughts come your way; direct them back to the Third Eye.

Practice the meditation for 10 to 20 minutes while saying in silent or loudly, "May I see and perceive clearly on each level and seek only the truth." Take a few moments after mediation before moving on with the rest activities of your day.

Meditation for Crown Chakra

The meditation for the seventh chakra should focus on bringing the energy from up through feet to all the other six chakras. Sit down on your knees with legs crossed and close your eyes. Imagine the energy on top of your head, and there is also a white light in the form of a ball that enlarges each time you inhale a deep breath. The energy will start coursing through you, and you might forget your physical being for some time as you focus on bringing the energy up to your crown.

You will also start to feel a slight tingle on your crown when the energy ball is large enough. At this point, imagine the energy is flowing to the rest of the body. After the mediation practice, you will feel a sigh of relief, and you will experience a strong connection between your body, mind, and spirit.

Chapter 2: Chakra Stones

Chakra stones are diverse types of stones in numerous colors that are used to support the chakra healing practice.

The human body has chakras with specific colors each. When these chakras are not functioning as required, their colors will change.

Chakra stones are intended to assist your chakras in finding balance within you as well as the greater sense of peace and harmony. Chakra can misalign because they are often described as spinning energy wheels. They can also collapse into a sluggish turn or spin too fast.

Losing the balance of one of the chakra is often felt because each one of them corresponds to a particular part of us either spiritually, emotionally, physically, and mentally.

Chakra stones will come in handy to enable you to pre-empt such a situation as you learn more about how to use them to deal with such a situation. Each chakra as we had learned earlier has its own color representation. Each chakra also has its own symptoms of problems, and it's important you observe carefully which problem or illness is recurring. Upon clear knowledge of which chakra has a problem, it's important you choose the exact chakra stone that will heal, clear and balance that chakra.

Chakra stones can be chosen from a variety of crystal in any number because the ultimate goal is to find the vital equilibrium to help your chakra function well. If you happen to collect and keep precious stones for any other purpose, and not for healing properties, you might be shocked to learn you have some pieces that are a solution to one or more of your chakras problem.

Chakras stones are all the same and serve an equal purpose and it doesn't matter whether one is more expensive or rare or naturally beautiful than the other stones. If you have the right color, you are good to align your chakra as required.

Chakra Stone for Root

The right chakra stones that will help you to align your root chakra are the red and black ones. You will feel more grounded, solid, stable, and proud of yourself.

The recommended chakra stones for root chakra include Ruby, Black Obsidian, Hematite, Smoky Quartz, Red Jasper, Jet, Black Onyx, Fire Opal, Bloodstone and Red Garnet.

You are required to place any type of the above-mentioned stones for your root chakra just close to your groin and between your thighs. Think about the color red or black as you think about your more solid core, a stronger passion for all things, a happier and a stronger foundation.

Chakra Stone for Sacral Chakra

When your Sacral Chakra is overactive, you will experience frequent frustrations and the underactive second chakra will make you feel like you lack joy.

There are various chakra stones that will help you align your sacral chakra and they include Orange Calcite, Orange Aventurine, Tiger's Eye, Orange Jasper, Carnelian, Sunstone, Fire Opal, Tangerine Quartz and Brown Citrine.

Once your Sacral Chakra is aligned, you will be inspired, motivated, and get the excitement that you need.

Chakra Stone for Solar Plexus Chakra

When your Solar Plexus Chakra is aligned, you will have new brilliant ideas. The right Chakra Stones to use for you to heal your Solar Plexus are the yellow gemstones like Yellow Jasper, Amber, Golden Calcite, Rutilated Quartz, Moonstone, Citrine, Fire Opal, Pyrite and Topaz.

Aligning your Solar Plexus Chakra will enable you to feel goal-oriented, inspired, and confident. To use these stones on your Solar Plexus Chakra, lie down and face up, place the stone 2 inches apart from the position of your belly. Think of the color yellow in your mind and an extremely bright sunny.

Chakra Stones for Heart Chakra

When your chakra is aligned, you are more open and relaxed and you are ready to accept new relationships, maintain healthy relationships, ready to forgive and feel love.

To help you with aligning your heart chakra, use the following recommended Chakra stones: Green Aventurine, Emerald, Peridot, Rhodonite, Green Tourmaline, Rose Quartz, Green Moss Agate, Pink Tourmaline, Jade, Ruby, Chrysoprase, Malachite, Rhodochrosite, and Watermelon Tourmaline.

You will become positive again, strengthen your relationships, and radiate love.

Chakra Stones for Throat Chakra

When your Throat Chakra is not stable, you will find that you are having difficulties expressing your thoughts, leading to miscommunication and frustration.

Choosing blue chakra stones will help you stabilize your Throat Chakra. They include Blue aragonite, Lapis Lazuli, Angelite, Blue Apatite, Blue Calcite, Turquoise, Aquamarine, Sodalite, Blue Sapphire, and Blue Lace Agate.

When your throat chakra is aligned, communicating, and expressing yourself becomes easy.

Chakra Stones for Third Eye

When your Third Eye is misaligned, you will be closed off to new ideas, and you will feel like you are incapable of trusting anybody and your intuition will be out of sorts.

Some of the chakra stones you will use to stabilize your Third Eye Chakra are Amethyst, Fluorite, Azurite, Blue Aventurine, Lapis Lazuli, Lolite, Celestite, Angelite and Sugilite.

When your Third Eye is aligned, you will have a stronger intuition, clearer mind, and your ability to resolve your issues and problems will be enhanced.

Chakra Stones for The Crown Chakra

Having unstable Crown Chakra will make you feel stressed and unable to think clearly. You will feel lost, and most or all aspects of your life will look uncertain. You will feel like you are living a life without direction or purpose.

The following chakra stones will significantly help, and they include White Topaz, Moonstone, Blue Opal, Amethyst, Selenite, Blue Sapphire, White Calcite, and Clear Quartz.

To heal your Crown Chakras, simply use the above stones by putting them on your head top and thinking about violet or white light. Your life will be full of light and purpose. You will also have a positive perspective from the setbacks that you might experience, and you will be able to work towards achieving your life goals.

How to Understand You Are Opening Your Chakras

Every thought, feeling, emotion, and experience we have is about our energy system and chakras. Because we use chakras all the time, it is important we pay keen attention to all the aspects of our living to understand when we are opening our chakras and also when its imbalanced or blocked. For instance, if I have controlling tendencies but I am highly energetic and motivated, it means I have imbalanced chakras and I need to work on it for it to stabilize. Below is a brief summary to help you understand the behavior of each chakra when they are open:

Understanding Open First Chakra-Root

Your physical body will be healthy, you will have a basic sense of safety and security, and you will feel grounded. You will have healthy feet, bones, weight, adrenal glands, colon, and elimination. The functioning of your practical side of life will be excellent.

Understanding Open Second Chakra-Sacral Chakra

You will have balanced sexuality, good life energy, open to change, healthy urinary, and reproductive systems. You will also experience joy, and you will neither have overactive nor underactive second chakra.

Understanding Open Third Chakra-Solar Plexus

When your third chakra is open, you will have the ability to achieve your goals in the physical world. You will have a sense of self-worth. There will have a healthy immune system, digestion, muscle system, and adrenals. You will not have any major allergy issues.

Understanding Open Fourth Chakra- Heart

You will have compassion for others when this chakra is open. You will also be able to maintain healthy relationships, have a sense of emotional satisfaction, feel connected to nature, and forgive others. You will show kindness to yourself and others. You will have healthy lungs, hands, arms, thymus, and heart.

Understanding Open Fifth Chakra- Throat

When this chakra is open, you will have the ability to express yourself and your own truth. You will be able to listen, have creative expression, have healthy mouth, ears, neck, shoulders, sinuses, nose, and thyroid voice.

Understanding Open Sixth Chakra- Third Eye

You will have intellect balanced with other intelligence attributes like good focus, insight, excellent memory, intuition, and be able to see the 'big picture.' You will have healthy eyes, vision, hypothalamus, and pituitary gland.

Understanding Seventh Chakra Health-Crown

If your seventh chakra is open, you will feel a sense of connection to greater purpose and power; you will feel wiser, have inner peace, greater developed consciousness, acceptance of others and have the stable mentality. You will have a healthy pineal gland and cerebral cortex.

How to Open Root Chakras (Red)

One of the most efficient ways to open your chakra is by first grounding yourself, meaning you should attach yourself with the ground. To achieve this, adjust your feet shoulder-width to stay apart, move your pelvis forward as you slightly bend your knees. Distribute your eight evenly by keeping your body balanced. Sit cross-legged after grounding yourself and attach your index finger to your thump in a peaceful motion.

Focus on the root chakra and imagine a closed red flower with extremely powerful energy glowing it and opens displaying four petals that are filled with energy. Contract, hold, and release perineum breath for twenty to thirty minutes. This should help you open your root chakra.

How to Open Sacra Chakra

To open your second chakra, start by sitting on your knees in an upright posture or straightened back. Rest your hands in your lap and ensure the inside of your palms is facing upwards. Touch the back fingers of your right hand with your left hand, meaning it will be underneath your right hand. Attach the thumps of both hands together. Focus on the chakra and the part it represents, below the navel. Silently, chant the word "VAM" while gently breathing. Do this for about 30 minutes or more until you feel completely relaxed. This practice will clear your mind and ensure your sacral chakra is open.

How to Open Solar Plexus Chakra

Sit on your knees in an upright posture. Place your hand before the stomach just below the upper abdomen where solar plexus chakra is located. Place your fingers together with your thumps closed and point them to the direction away from you. Focus on your chakra and its location on your body. Clearly chant the word "RAM" while continuing to think about chakra and what it means, including how it affects the different aspects of life. Practice this process until you are relaxed and feel clean.

How to Open Your Heart Chakra

Sit down with your legs crossed. Attach your index fingers to your thumbs in your both hands. Place your right hand below your breastbone and your left hand on your left knee. Maintain that position for 20 minutes or more as you think about your heart chakra and what it exists in your body, at the center of your chest. Chant the word "YAM" silently as you continue to relax and think about your heart chakra. Continue with the practice until you feel clean. You will have a feeling of great compassion after few moments after practicing this process and opening your heart chakra.

How to Open Your Throat Chakra

Again, start by sitting on your knees. Cross all your fingers insides and leave the thumps. Attach your thumps together at the top. Focus on your throat chakra and what it represents, at the base of your throat. Silently but clearly, chant the word "HAM" while continuing to think about your throat chakra and how it affects your life. Do this for 10 to 15 minutes, and you will have a feeling of relaxation and cleanliness.

How to Open Your Third Eye Chakra

Sit cross-legged. Place your hands below your breastbone. Point your middle finger away from you while touching their tops. Focus on the third eye chakra and the part it represents, the center of your eyes. Silently chant the word "AUM" or "OM." Allow your body to relax naturally as you continue to think about your chakra and how it affects your life. Practice for 20 minutes or more until you feel clean and/or intensified to focus and come up with brilliant ideas to achieve your goals.

How to Open Your Crown Chakra

Sit with your legs crossed. Cross your fingers together except for the little fingers which you should touch them against each other at the top and let them point up and in the opposite direction away from you. The right thumb should be placed at the top of the left thumb. Focus on the crown chakra, and what it represents, the top of your head.

General Guidelines to Help You Know Which Chakra to Open

Step 1: Know Your Chakras

One of the very important step while preparing to open your chakras is to know them. Each one of the chakras has several distinct qualities that are different from one another. That also means the practice of opening them is very different. We might feel scattered or exhausted when our chakras are imbalanced or blocked. We might also feel ill. Know what each chakra represents, the signs that they are either blocked or imbalanced so that you can know how to take care of them as required.

Step 2: Establish the Level of Need

Because you have a total of seven well-known chakras, identify which one you want to handle first. It is sometimes difficult to identify which one needs help than the others. That is because when one is misaligned, it affects all the others. There are several signs that you can look up to identify the most problematic chakra. One of the first steps is to take the chakra test by analyzing all your body parts and check which one has more problems.

Also, check whether you can identify physical pain in the corresponding area represented by a particular chakra. You can also check what is happening in your life and identify problematic issues such as financial problems, safety issues, relationship issues, an emotional roller-coaster or lack of motivation, etc. You can also visit a professional chakra energy healing expert or a close friend or colleague who is energy-conscious.

Step 3: Activate the Energy to Open Your Chakra

At this stage, you have identified the problematic chakra. No start planning how to open that chakra, and it's important that you also think of it as a plan to restore your chakra. By opening that chakra, you are also balancing the flow (both inflow and outflow) of your energy; you are also increasing its state and variations awareness. The main principle used by professional healers and most energy-conscious people is the idea of balancing or balance while opening your chakras.

Some of the practices that you will need to use while opening your chakra include breathing exercise, physical activity with the main focus on the particular location of that chakra. Take part in a healing session (find a professional healer or energy-conscious person), use chakra connection techniques or massages (also known as 'self-healing hands-on technique), meditation technique focusing on that particular chakra location).

While practicing any of these techniques to heal your chakra, it is important to be aware that other things might come up in the process. When opening your chakra, remember there are issues that made it block or become unbalanced in the first place. These things are more likely to come up, and this is your chance to deal with them consciously. Always take care of yourself by ensuring you are focused and aware and mindful of all what is happening as you open your chakras.

Check which practice resonates with you or makes the most sense when choosing the most appropriate chakra opening technique. Evaluate whether you need a meditative or physical practice. Your availability will also determine the type of practice to pick, you might only have a few minutes, or you might also be able to schedule an hour or more

Chapter 3: Breathing Techniques to Help Your Chakra Remain Open

Most effective techniques, such as belly breathing involve the use of your belly to pass more energy and awareness. It will improve your general wellness and health if you learn and master this technique.

You will also learn it's not just the breathing that is important but remembering how to breathe well. The focus should be on the intent to enhance the benefits that come with using breathing techniques the right way. During the practice, it is important to become conscious of the breath, which is equally vital for your mind, physical body, and soul to be optimized.

Belly breathing is a helpful technique to enable you to maximize your health, increase your energy, and bring more consciousness to your body.

What Belly Breathing Technique Involve?

Attach your index fingers together and your thumbs together as well and place them below your navel or in the second chakra area just above the pubic area. Imagine feeling this area as you breathe. Breathing into the belly will make you feel fuller and deeper. It will also help in giving your breath the appropriate direction. It is easier to breathe into your belly while you are either lying or standing up. You can also practice while sitting, but it is not easy because you might fill your chest instead of your belly.

Focus on your breathing to make sure you are filling your belly and not your chest.

It is normal and common to imagine your breath flowing from downwards to upwards moving through your chest to the crown and out of our heads. It is the reason why we lift our chest to allow the air inside our lungs and fill them while breathing deeply. We often calm our nervous system and reduce stress and anxiety.

However, by breathing up and out, all your good energy or prana is exhaled out into the air. You will not benefit in strengthening your chakras if you breathe out. Nevertheless, it's ok if your chakras are already strong and well balanced, you can then choose to breathe out.

NOTE: For belly breathing, imagine and do the reverse. Instead of inhaling and breathing out, draw your breath inwards and downwards then draw it deep into your belly.

In some cases, there are people who are deep chest breather and others who are belly breather. If you categorize yourself as a deep chest breather, try minimizing your chest lifting. Allow your belly to collapse as you exhale. It might not be easy at first, but doing more practices will help you master the technique. It is also ok for you to lift your chest but make sure your belly is moving fast.

Some people have a tendency to hold their bellies, especially when they are influenced by the desire to look thin. They unknowingly hold strong emotions within the abdomen area, which later becomes the second chakra problems. The holding of unacceptable feelings is placed deep in the core of our beings. It is these denied and unacknowledged emotions that later come to haunt us in the form of diseases.

It might be difficult, fearful, or uncomfortable for people who have suffered trauma to practice belly breathing, and it is important for those facing difficulty to seek professional counseling.

Steps to Enable You Practice Belly Breathing

1. First, breathe in and draw the breath deep and down into the belly. To get more focus, watch your belly rise. You can also focus on your hands you had placed on the belly rise as well. If you continue practicing more, you will not need to place your hands in your belly, but if you enjoy the practice while they are there, it's ok with it.

2. When exhaling and your hands and belly retract downwards towards your spine, make sure you are holding your breath in your belly. Don't allow your prana to flow out and gather the life force into your being.

3. To help you fill your belly quick, imagine and picture it in your mind as if you are filling a store with each breath you inhale and also imagine exhaling as you keep your remaining breath in your abdomen.

And these are all the necessary steps you need to learn about the belly breathing techniques. Always make sure you have at least done 10 breaths to recover fully. If you are used to yoga breathing, belly breathing might be a challenge because you are used to inhale a little amount of oxygen. You can just try to breathe the normal way and practice belly breathing as the days pass.

Practicing belly breathing at least once or twice a day, especially when you feel your body and mind is dragging. This practice will make you gain more energy, and you will feel a change.

Sending Your Energy to Specific Chakra Areas after Gathering In The Belly

Once you have learned and mastered how to gather your breath or energy or prana in your belly, the next step is to distribute in other parts of your body.

This time around, you will inhale and gather your breath or prana deep into the belly and as you exhale, direct it to other parts of the body that you are seeking to heal and imagine it as you practice.

It is especially crucial to practice energy distribution if you are ill, broken, or stuck. If you have a problem with your throat, for instance, you will send the life force energy to the throat, and it won't take before you notice changes. If you wish to get more feelings of compassion and love, direct your breath over your heart and your down your breastbone and up your throat as you exhale.

Also, when any part of your body is stuck say, your shoulders, or hip, inhale the air deep into your belly and send energy or prana to your stick shoulder or hip as you exhale. It won't take a long time before you experience changes.

It might look difficult to visualize how to hold your breath in your belly and to send it in the form of energy to different parts of the body, but with practice, it will become easier. Where the breath and mind goes, the energy and prana go, that is the basic rule when practicing breathing techniques to heal your chakra.

You can also use the following breathing technique in steps to help heal your prana.

1. Sit comfortably, cross your legs, ensure your lips are gently sealed and breathe using your nose. Put your palms together and keep them raised above your head.

2. Draw as much breath as possible as you inhale deeply into your belly. You can choose to close your eyes or open them wide but either way, imagine drawing as much light as possible as it passes through your eyes, on top of your head, your face, and ears.

3. Whenever your lungs are full, they are also full of prana. Close your eyes, whether they were open or not, and focus your awareness between your eyes. Form a sphere of concentrated and bright light at your point of focus, the area between your eyebrows. You might experience lightning flashes or sparks; however, you should never lose focus and continue to focus and remain comfortable.

4. Watch the light dissolve to other body parts that require healing or balancing as you

exhale. Perform the practice at least 10 or 15 times or more.

Our body is full of energy that we breathe all the time. Besides coming from the air we breathe, it also comes from the food we eat, the water we drink, and from sunlight. Practicing these breathing techniques allow us to utilize the vast amount of prana in our body and heal our chakras. We also heal our spiritual being, our souls, and our minds. We prevent any physical discomfort or illness when we help heal our chakras through these breathing techniques. We also give purpose to our lives, live peacefully with others, make wise decisions, and have excellent relationships.

Chapter 4: Nutrition and Chakras System

Eating is a powerful action and one of the ways in which we breathe in our prana and use for healing. Taking food is also one of the most integral activities in our lives that enable us to survive and live. Whether you are a nutritionist or not, you understand that foods are conduits to human growth, especially if the right food is taken.

Each chakra has a special nutritional diet that needs to be taken, and we will discuss each one of them:

Nutritional Food for Root Chakra

The root chakra is an excellent place to release fear around feelings of dishonest and eating. Over-eating or under-eating might make you feel scattered. Your root chakra's work is to enable you to feel grounded so that you have a clear mind to make wise decisions and relate well with those around your life.

The best nutritional food that will enable you to be grounded and boost the purpose of your root chakra include minerals, proteins, red-colored foods, medicinal and edible mushrooms, and root vegetables.

Eating with other community members will also help your root chakra. You can also dialogue with your body to enable you to honor your body's instinct on which of these chakra works best to heal your chakra.

Nutritional Food for Sacral Chakra

The sacral chakra is the exact opposite of the first chakra. While the root chakra keeps us grounded and stable, the sacral chakra opens up to the movement and flow. When you are having problems with your creativity or expressing yourself, "You are not going with the flow." Eating the right food will help your sacral chakra continue with the flow.

The sacral chakra foods include seeds, tropical fruits, orange-colored foods, fats, and oils (omega-3s is one of the best), nuts, and fish.

While eating, it is important to pay attention to your senses.

Nutritional Food for Solar Plexus Chakra

Solar Plexus gives us the power that we need to give us the drive to achieve our goals and make wise decisions. We can also go into overdrive, and in this situation; we are bound to lose power.

However, you can harness your power and energy to be optimal by looking at the type of foods that you should take. Eat food that will assist you in sustaining your energy and try to eat them as frequently as possible.

The foods that will help solar plexus in serving its purpose include whole grains, yellow-colored nutritional foods, fiber, legumes, fiber, and complex carbohydrates.

Avoid food that will weaken your body, such as artificial sweeteners, sugars, soft drinks, and avoid drinking excessive alcoholic beverages.

Nutritional Food for Heart Chakra

The heart chakra gives us the ability to give love and compassion. Your heart energy will dry if this chakra is not in balance.

Food for love and compassion include foods rich in chlorophyll, sprouts, vegetables, any green-colored nutritional food, and raw foods.

The heart chakra will also flourish if you share foods with others, express gratitude for feeding yourself and infuse love into the water we are drinking and the food that we are eating during meals.

Nutritional Food for Throat Chakra

The throat chakra is responsible for illuminating our truth and genuineness. It is also the pathway to our food and where several activities take place, including chewing, swallowing, breathing, and talking.

The foods that will help your throat chakra in communicating and telling the truth include fruits, juices, sea plants, sauces, and soups.

We should also not create an imbalance in our throat chakra, especially when sating our food choices—for example, avoid saying "yes" to some food choices when we really mean "no."

Nutritional Food for The Third Eye Chakra

The third eye is the center of our intuition, inspiration, imagination, and insight. Listening to this intuition nourishes our center. We can lose sight if we allow our intellect to override our intuition.

The foods that help our third eye and stimulate our intuitive center include herbal tea, blueberries, and blackberries.

 When your third chakra is unbalanced or is already in an overdrive situation, avoid food or beverages such as dark chocolate, alcohol, and coffee. These foods will stimulate and keep your moods and mind on overdrive.

Nutritional Food for Your Crown Chakra

Crown Chakra connects us all to life. Choosing to eat is a very satisfying form of interconnection when you feel severed from bigger things like the human race, planet, your community, or the cosmos. Eating the right nutritional food for crown chakra will enable you to get a deeper meaning when thinking about life.

Food that helps you with your crown chakra includes copal, juniper, sage, frankincense, and myrrh. Also feed your crowd chakra with clean air, unconditional love and moon-and-sun light.

Foods are excellent symbols of connection that will enable you to connect with deeper and sacred aspects of life.

Chakras Endocrine System and the Immune System

The endocrine system is a chemical messenger where internal glands produce hormones directly into the bloodstream during the circulatory process. The internal glands are part of different organs in our body, and the endocrine system helps in regulating all the organs in our bodies.

All Seven Chakras control different glands:

- Root Chakra – control adrenal gland

The adrenal is found at the top of the kidneys that produce hormones, including adrenaline, which is responsible for stimulating the "flight or fight" response. The adrenaline gland is also responsible for root chakra's survival drive, which directly ties to the base.

- Sacral Chakra – control reproductive system-including ovaries

The ovaries are responsible for controlling egg creation, sexual development, and controlling progesterone and estrogens. The drives of the sacral chakra mirror the ovaries' potential for life. The sacral chakra also links with the energies of the ovaries.

- Solar Plexus – controls the pancreas

The pancreas is responsible for hormones like insulin, which helps in our digestive systems.

Overstimulating the solar plexus chakra with things like excess blood sugar can cause various problems which can lead to diseases like diabetes. Under stimulating your solar plexus can lead to ulcers.

- Heart Chakra – controls the Heart and Thymus

The thymus is responsible for producing lymphocytes, which is an important part used for digestion and the immune system. Because of this quality, the thymus is referred to as one of the vital healing properties of your fourth or heart chakra.

- Throat Chakra – controls thyroid

The thyroid is contained on either side of the larynx, which is part of the throat chakra. The thyroid produces the hormone called thyroxine, which is responsible for controlling the rate of food conversion by the body into useful energy.

In this particular area, the throat chakra is dominant. The rate of metabolism is governed by the thyroid.

- Third Eye-Controls the Pituitary Gland

The pituitary gland is near the skull base and is responsible for releasing hormones that influence the chemistry of our body. The third eye spiritual energies are reflected by the pituitary glands and their influence on our whole body.

The third eye and pituitary gland work together in the body.

- Crown Chakra-control pineal gland

Pineal produces melatonin hormones and lies deep within our brain.

This hormone mirrors the relationship between the crown chakra and other chakras because it

affects all the other glands in your endocrine
system.

Crown chakra and pineal gland are part of the
determinants of the entire system.

Chapter 5: Chakra Cleansing Meditation

There are different meditation techniques you can use to cleanse your chakras. Our chakras are sometimes filled with negative or unnecessary thoughts and feelings, and if they are not cleansed, they might get out of control and even lead to illnesses, depression, addictive behaviors like drugs and alcoholism. You will also not be able to be productive or effective in whatever you are trying to accomplish. It is important you take important steps and practice any form of techniques that will cleanse your chakras for a healthy and productive life.

1st Example of Chakra Cleansing Meditation

1. Sit comfortably in a leveled space or ground. Inhale deeply and relax as you exhale. Relax as you perform the practice as you connect with the environment as well.

2. Listen careful to sounds inside you, these sounds might be as a result of cleansing done through your chakras.

3. Release everything that you don't need and
    throw away into the earth and be aware of
    your space and the rising and falling of your
    breath.

4. Breathe down to your roots, allow the roots
    to connect down to the ground. Let your
    root chakra take everything it needs and put
    all those into your imagination.

5. Allow the energy flow to your sacral chakra,
    breathe deeply, and exhale comfortably and
    gently. Continue to your other chakras
    including Solar plexus, Throat, Heart, Third
    Eye, and Crown Chakras. Take time and
    allow all these chakras to fully cleanse
    themselves and get rid of everything they
    don't need.

6. Continue with this form of cleaning
    meditation for at least 20 minutes or more
    and only stop when you feel your chakras
    are fully cleansed.

Heart Cleansing and Forgiveness meditation

1. Start by sitting with a straight back, breathe
    in, and exhale gently. Focus on the moment.

2. Evaluate whether your consciousness is filled with a sincere desire to cleanse. Use the following affirmations which are

3. "My true self show me the truth of who I am."

4. Allow yourself to get rid of all negative thoughts and feelings. Be true to all the feelings you have and get rid of those that you don't need.

5. Think of any person or people that you might have had negative thoughts towards, and it's good to start with those people who you carry the greatest resentment towards them.

6. Invite the imaginations of the reasons why you hold resentment towards a particular person or group of people. It might be because of their "controlling nature" if he is your boss. Or it might also be because of the "abusive nature" of a colleague you don't like. Whichever the case, don't judge them, imagine if you have similar behaviors in you or not.

7. Think about the way or how you felt mistreated.

8. Pretend that person who offends you or mistreats you is in the room with you, imagine them saying what they are used to say or annoy you as they usually do while you are watching them. Allow them in your imaginations to continue over and over until you feel their behavior or utterances are not affecting you anymore.

9. Understand that whichever the way they mistreat and abuse, you are just words and negative behaviors and look beyond and cleanse these thoughts.

10. This form of cleansing meditation should take you at least 5 minutes or more.

11. You will be able to feel less or not bothered by those who you feel you dislike and whichever manner they continue treating you, you will tend to treat them with compassion without holding any grudges or negative feelings towards them.

Cleansing Using Sunlight Purification Technique

1. This requires you to perform on a sunny day or during the day. The light serves as an awareness of your pure consciousness. Go outside, stand, and raise your hands.
2. Allow the light from the sun to flow into your crown head and distribute it to other parts of the body. Imagine the bright sunlight cleansing your chakras as it pours through the locations of the body parts representing all the seven chakras.
3. Also, imagine this light pouring continuously, and the cleansing been performed is thoroughly and endlessly.
4. Feel the chakras been fed with positive thoughts. For instance, feel the heart chakra been filled with unconditional love. Your throat filled with excellent expression and communication power.
5. Also imagine and feel the light cleansing all your body organs, tissues, and muscles from one part of one chakra locations to all the other locations.

6. Perform the sunlight meditation cleansing for the next 5 minutes or more or until you feel you have cleansed yourself.

A Heart Chakra Mediation Technique

You will start by finding a place or ground that is relaxed and comfortable and with no possibility of disturbances. Sit and make sure your back is straight, breathe using your nose and exhale through your mouth. Inhale and exhale in this particular for at least 5 to 10 minutes or more and relax your body as you do this. Imagine drawing up green energy towards your heart via your body, starting at the base of your body and up to your heart and out. Imagine that green energy becoming brighter and bigger as you inhale and exhale and picture it as a bright huge green ball.

Focus yourself tuning on giving love and compassion to yourself and others while allowing the green energy radiate through your body and focus on performing these meditation techniques for at least 5 minutes or more.

Present Moment Focus and Cleansing

This form of cleansing is important, especially if you wish to get rid of the numerous problems that you are experiencing in your life.

1. Close your eyes and inhale deeply while exhaling gently.
2. Think about everything in your life, your negative thoughts, what people think about you and your thoughts about who you are or who wish to be and put that aside.
3. Take out all your past and observe the present, all the opportunities available and hat you wish to do and perform.
4. If you sense some straining in some thoughts such as what you want to happen or if they are unrealistic, get rid of them and let them go.
5. Your mindset is now clear, be open to thoughts, and allow yourself to be filled with positive and clear thinking.

Use Unifying Phrase Meditation

Most of the human suffering comes from the brain and meditation allows us to relax and be open to ourselves in getting read of negative or stressful thoughts and allow us to be filled with positive energies and thoughts. The use of unifying meditation is a different form of affirmation that tends to paint over a suffering mind and thoughts. Unifying phrase enables you to completely shift your attention from bad and negative thoughts and energies in your being to prepare a doorway to the positive and fulfilling thoughts.

Shifting your thoughts and mindset will enable you to easily get rid of unwanted thinking and memory and replace it with good and positive energies and memories.

Start by closing your eyes or leave them open and inhale deeply and exhale smoothly while uttering the following unifying phrases.

"I allow accepting everything the way it is at this moment."

"I am conscious and aware of everything around me."

"I choose peace."

"I am at peace with my creator."

The unifying meditation can also be spiritual and serve the purpose of choosing to side with your creator and everything that is on the side of good and positivity.

Chapter 6: Tips to Balance Your Chakra

If you wish to bring more joy and peace into your life, balancing and aligning your chakra is the way to go. When the chakras are not in balance, our mental and physical health is out of balance as well. We experience many other bad experiences like fear, depression, worry, and even falling sick. There are several tips that you can use to help you with balancing your chakras. They are simple and easy to understand, and they include:

- Colors

It is important for you to understand different colors representing your chakras. Your intuition should guide you on which colors to wear. Each chakra resonates with a particular color, and since all the chakras are different energy centers which have a specific frequency, you must match them with their respective color to similar frequency. When balancing any chakra, for instance, if you are practicing to balance the root chakra, try your best to wear red color whether it's your outer clothes or undergarment. You can also burn red candles around you while practicing chakra. The red color will help filter your chakra's color and assist you in readdressing the balance of your root chakra.

- Food

The diet you eat is very important when it comes to balancing your chakra. There are specific foods for a particular chakra, and it's vital for us to have this knowledge. Also, you should try to match the color of the food with the chakra you are trying to balance. For instance, in addition to eating the right diet for your root chakras such as root vegetables, protein, and minerals, add colored food to your diets such as radishes, tomatoes, pomegranates, watermelon, and even peppers. Watch the color of any other chakra that you might be trying to balance.

- Spend More Time in Nature

To absorb the healing of nature, it is also important you do your best to get the help of healing energy from nature through means such as walking barefoot and sitting in the grass. You can also perform your chakra balancing techniques in the outdoor setting in the grass, beside the river or trees. This will assist you in bringing more joy and peace into your life and keeping you grounded.

Having a beautiful garden in your compound is a helpful idea. Also, add plants and flowers in your home to help with the chakra balancing.

- Practice Breathing Deeply More Regularly

Breathing deeply is one of the major techniques of restoring your chakras.

During your free moments or when practicing meditation to help balance your chakra, learn how to breathe deeply, direct your breath to different chakra parts when exhaling and letting awareness to settle in your chakras.

- Sound

Just like chakra colors, our energy centers or chakras resonate to particular musical notes as well

For Root=C

Solar Plexus=D

Heart=F

Throat=G

Third Eye=A

Crown=B

Listening to the notes above with intent to balance the chakra it represents will help you stimulate that specific chakra or energy center. If classical music is closely available, they are very good in helping align unbalanced chakras.

- Essential Oils

Essential oils are also a great booster when it comes to balancing your chakras. You can either apply them by inhaling or directly on your skin all over your body or body parts. However, if you wish to apply directly to your skin, use a suitable carrier oil and dilute your essential oil before rubbing it against your skin.

- Practice Creative Visualization

The first step is to clear your mind to enable you to have a successful visualization. After clearing your mind, do your best to visualize images that signify love and happiness.

Visualize a heart blessing your entire chakras one at a time or a flower opening. Also, visualize cleansing each and every energy center, with relevant sound, color, and frequency.

- Practice Toning with Your Own Voice

During your free time, exercise using your voice to come up with stimulating tones that will help in balancing your chakras. Start by placing your hands in the chakra that is unbalanced and start making sound and make sure it's the deepest tone possible. Start with low tone and gradually increase your pitch as you continue. With regular practice, you will eventually get the right pitch for you, and you will notice your unbalanced chakra responding to your tone. You that correct tune throughout the week or day until your center of energy feel more balanced.

- Practice Gratitude

Your vibrational frequency will rise when you show gratitude towards yourself and others. Raised vibrations enable you to open your chakra, and you will start experiencing positive things in your life such as happiness, abundance, better relationships and have more peace within yourself, your life and with other people.

Also, do your best to connect and making friends, and if you are shy or fear other people, try your best to heal or balance your heart chakra and other chakras as well. Failing to correct your ability to strengthen your relationships or connect with others can affect your social or romantic life, and in worst situations, it can also affect your career success. Show gratitude to open your chakras and improve your social life and other positive things in life.

Other Chakra Balancing Tips Include

- Indulge your Mind

It is in the sacral chakra where you hold energies related to cravings and addiction. Avoid lacking discipline or restricting yourself too much. Go out for adventures or to chat up with friends or indulge with other fun activities. Always indulge yourself with consciousness while engaging in any activity, whether its food, alcohol, sex, or even social media.

- Unleash Your Creativity

Creativity is important for your emotional, physical, spiritual, and mental health. Everyone has creative skills, passion, or talent, and some people are yet to discover. Just do creative things to help grow yourself as a person and for your sacral chakra.

- Learn to Say "No" When Required

When you are empowered, your solar plexus is aligned. Say no and reject any activity or event that you feel is not fulfilling. Also, say no to negative habits or partnership that you feel are not fulfilling. Most of the things that make you waste your time are also responsible for weakening or unbalancing your solar plexus, which also hosts the energies of independence, motivation, and joy.

- Learn to Say "Thank you" and "Please"

When your feelings of kindness, acceptance, and generosity are harnessed, your heart chakra is well balanced. Learn the kind act of equally giving and receiving love for your heart chakra to balance. Learn to say simple words like 'thank you' or 'please'.

- Pay Attention to Your Dreams

Intuition speaks to us in various ways, and a dream is one of them. Ignoring your intuitive will make your third eye chakra to become blocked or imbalanced. Pay attention to your dreams, especially those that make great sense realistically to know how you have been guided. Keep note of the little messages over a period of time to get the big picture of what your soul is communicating to you through your dreams.

- Surrender Your Faith

Having the belief of the existence of a higher being might also help you to balance your crown chakra. You can also expand your crown chakra by affirming what or to whom the faith you have in.

- Prepare Journal

A healthy throat chakra requires you to be honest all the time. Be honest to yourself before coming to terms or been authentic to anybody else. Write down your exact feelings and the emotions that you are holding. Have all the thoughts that are running in your mind in a journal without fear or judgment. Don't try to be juicy in your journal and write everything as it is, and this will enable you to be honest with yourself and to others.

- Write a Letter

It is common for people to avoid hearing the truth from you or even wanting to hear your words. Do yourself a favor and get some of the issues off your chest and write them down. This will help you connect with your chakra and onto your paper. Getting issues out in the open will help you deal with them instead of holding them for no good reason. You are not going to send the letter anywhere, it's just for getting things out of your being, and you will see that it will be easier to deal with issues once you cease holding them in yourself.

- Activate Your Heart Chakra With Drumming

To help with the balancing of the heart chakra, drumming is one of the most helpful practices. Drumming has the ability to activate the heart chakra and therefore balancing lower chakra frequencies against higher chakra frequencies. Drum rhythms directly affect the heartbeats, according to scientific research. When drumming, your heart's pulse may slow down, speed up, or gradually tuned to the rhythm of the drum until a certain excellent synchronization is achieved.

- Perform Thorough Cleaning Around Your Home

Scheduling several hours or your day during the weekend or even weekdays if you have time just to perform cleaning chores around your home might be very helpful. Sometimes, chakra blockages can display in the form of disarray and untidiness in your house and rooms. Conducting a thorough cleaning will go a long way of helping you with your chakras and open a particular one or more of them.

- Colorful Light Candle Bath

Bathing is also part of balancing chakras, and it will boost your opening strategy if you light candles with colors that resonate with the chakra you wish to open. Colorful light bath technique will also clear your chakras as well. This will help you deal with various life aspects in a more meaningful manner.

- Sound Balancing

You can use sounds, and in chakra terms, they are either called seed or bija mantra. For instance, while balancing your throat chakra, repeat the mantra 'Ham' silently or aloud. Sound balancing practice requires you to combine with other balancing techniques like yoga or meditation.

- Watch Your Diet

Each chakra has its most appropriate diet. While opening your chakra, also ensure you are eating the right diet or foods that 'fuel' the chakras to balance or re-align itself. It is especially important to focus on eating the right diet of that particular chakra you are trying to open.

Chapter 7: Chakras Yoga

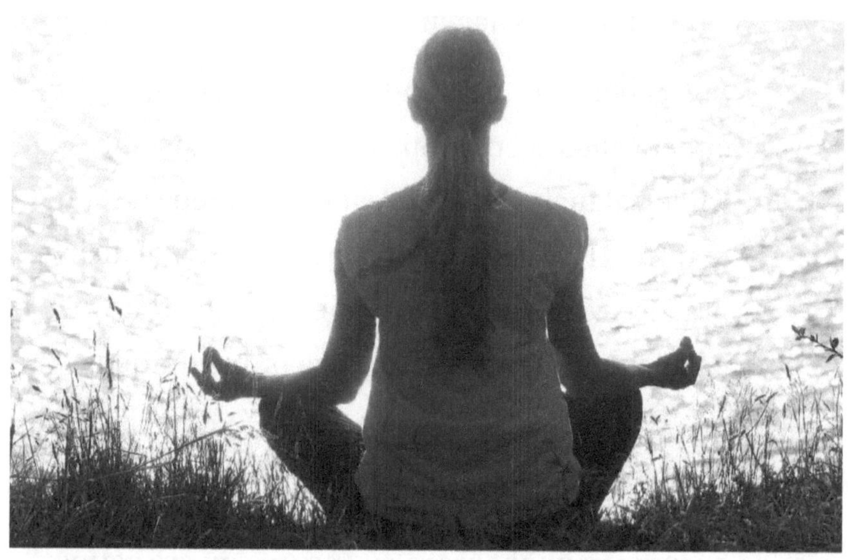

Yoga is one of the ways in which we can energize our chakras as well as align and balance them. By practicing yoga, we are also helping our spiritual, physical, and emotional attributes correspond to the chakra or frequency to get energized. Since chakras are also known to us as the 'spinning wheel,' it makes sense when we practice yoga because we release physical and emotional tension, which helps release the energy movement to flow freely. We will discuss specific yoga practices for each chakra:

Crow Pose

1. Stand and make sure your legs are three feet apart. Focus on your spine and feel it rising tall from the location of your pelvis. You will also feel the equal distribution of your weight between your feet on the surface of the ground or earth below you.

2. Squat slowly while maintaining the position of your feet on the earth. To help you maintain a straight posture, attach your palms together like a prayer posture, and place your elbows inside your two knees.

3. Inhale deeply and slowly into your abdomen, hold your breath for several minutes, and completely clear your lungs every time you exhale. Repeat this process for 20 to 30 minutes.

4. Release your hands, lie down and for a few minutes. Release the breath and let it continue to flow naturally. You will notice and feel prana moving through perineum physical area and other surrounding parts of your body, especially the coccyx and hips.

5. With more practice, you will master this root chakra yoga, and it will help you feel happy and worthy of your existence.

Yoga for Sacral Chakra

Pelvic Lifts

1. Lie down on the ground and ensure your spine is flat. Your head should also be on the ground as you face upwards. Feel your breath as it passes through your nostrils to your lungs, notice the movement of your rib cage as it goes up and down as you fill your lungs.

2. Bend the knees and let them point straight up in the sky. Ensure your souls that completely flat and close to your stretched arms on the ground. The palms of your hands should also touch the ground. You can also let your long middle finger touch your ankles to stay in the appropriate position.

3. Breathe in slowly and raise the pelvis to the highest level possible. Lift your spine gradually beginning with the lowermost

vertebrae. Then slowly move the spinal column.

4. Exhale as you slowly move your spine downwards again to its original position. You will the vertebra reconnect with each other as you go back to your previous position on the ground.

5. Repeat this process of lifting your pelvis up and down for at least 20 minutes. Ensure the movement is steady, smooth, slow, and meditative. Your breath should lead the movement, ensure your lungs are filled, your spine and arms fully stretched and you are fully exhaling as you move back down. Allow your spine to be responsible for moving the rest of the body. Also, visualize all your tension been erased by your breath. Do at least 3 to 6 lifts.

6. Trust that all the movements you are feeling are meant to heal and bring balance and harmony. You will notice some changes and your sacral chakra will be successfully healed if your practice this form of yoga.

Front Platform

1. Lie facing down with your stomach on the ground and toes pointing in the opposite direction or away from your head. Attach your palms to the ground as you bend your elbows.

2. Inhale and lift the body upwards as though you are doing a press up but with your toes still facing the opposite or backward direction.

3. Hold and stay in that upward position, start taking a deep breath and draw it into your abdomen and take long exhales as you push your breath out. Practice this process for at least 3 minutes is focusing on and feeling the prana flowing through the navel center.

This yoga practice will help you in healing and balancing your solar plexus.

Heart-Centering Meditation

1. Kneel and sit on your heels. Keep your spine in a straight position. Feel the flow of your breath as it fills your lungs as the diaphragm and solar plexus are lifted slightly.

2. Attach your middle fingers together as you extend your elbows sideways like flying wings and ensure your forearms stay parallel to the ground.

3. Lower your eyelids or close your eyes halfway and focus to gaze on your nose tip. The eye position is also widely used in other forms of yoga to focus, clear and silence the mind as well as activate pineal and pituitary glands.

4. You will hear vibrating inner voice in your mind with the mantra "Humme Hum Bram hum." You can also listen to the recorded version of this mantra while performing this type of yoga.

5. Extend your hands out slowly as you listen to this mantra. Inhale and exhale slowly

and feel as the prana flows through the center of your heart and radiating to your entire body.

Yoga for Throat Chakra

Camel

1. Kneel on the floor and ensure your legs are apart. Gently place your palms on your ankles as you lean backward while maintaining the same position.
2. Breath in an allow your heart to be lifted upwards as your thighs and hips press forward.
3. During exhaling, draw your shoulders towards each other so that your heart opens more deeply. Place your hands on your back to make the exhaling process much easier.
4. Focus on your throat while breathing deeply and continue moving the hips forward to allow the sternum to open up.
5. Drop your head backward to its original position and comfortably return your hands in the ankle.

6. Relax and allow prana to heal your throat as it produces silent inward vibrating sound "hmmmmmmmmm" every time you exhale. Release the sound out and continue this process for at least three minutes or more.

7. Successful performance of this chakra will allow you to make conscious choices and communicate authentic expressions that come from our true sense.

Yoga for Third Eye Chakra

Guru Pranam

1. To start this yoga pose, sit on your heels, and sit in an upright position. Inhale and feel prana arriving with every breath you take. You can use a firm pillow or blankets if you have difficulty sitting on your heels.

2. Extend your arms towards the ground as you comfortably spread your knees. Maintain the elongation of your spine by placing your forehead on the ground ahead and moving your lower back.

3. Focus on the vertebrae that are between the shoulders to enable the opening of the heart by melting that area.

4. Attach your palms together and visualize light as you inhale and exhale fully. Also, relax and let the force of gravity take control as well. Practice this yoga for at least 5 minutes or more.

5. Place your arms on the ground and gently lift your torso starting with the lowermost spine and rise up vertebra by vertebra and finish by lifting your head up. Before standing up, take a rest for few minutes or lie on your back.

6. After practicing this type of yoga, you will feel the change and discover that you can easily use logic and make excellent decisions.

Yoga for Crown Chakra

Guru Prasad

1. Sit on your heels and feel your spinal column been filled with light and rise up the

column. Take time to breathe in and feel as the prana flows through your breath.

2. Using your hands, make a bowl-shaped structure, and place your palms in front of your heart and face them up towards the sky. The bowl's purpose is to receive invisible light.

3. Place your upper arms against your rib cage. Feel the gifts from the universe been poured into your hands. The gifts will come one after the blessings come to you in a similar manner. Feel the presence of the infinite universe as you practice this yoga.

4. Focus on your nose tip and lower eyelid to leave just a small opening in your eyes. The focus will help you to open your third eye, and your optic nerve is also stimulated with the pineal gland. However, as you continue with your meditation, you are free to close the eyes to enable you to focus more on your third eye.

5. Take long, deep breaths and exhale completely while allowing your heart to

open for the feeling of love and compassion to penetrate through it.

6. Also, open yourself so that you can receive blessings in the form of many aspects, including consciousness and infinite universe.

7. Practice this form of mediation for at least 3 minutes. You can take more time if you feel you need it to heal your crown chakra completely.

8. Our consciousness will blossom if we allow the free flow of prana and healing of our crown chakra.

Malasana Yoga Pose

Squat and attach your palms together, breathe in deeply, hold for 30 seconds, and then exhale smoothly. Tuck the toes of your both feet and rest your chest on your knees as you practice this yoga pose. Don't lift your toes to get them out of the ground because it will disrupt your connection with the earth. This pose will help bring your being close to the earth, and the energy of the earth is felt through the feet while performing this practice.

Uttanasana

Stand up, fold your arms together by touching your right elbow with your left palm and doing the same with the left palm and touch your left elbow. Rest your folded hands on your head crown and then lean and bend forward at your waist with your folded arms and hands still intact. Ease your mind while practicing this yoga. This will enable us to find calmness and our center. It also releases tension from our entire back.

Mountain Pose

It is a chakra yoga practice that only involves standing up like a tree and feeling the support of the earth. This pose allows you to focus on the present moment and help us feel centered. Also, practice this yoga on the ground or grass to help you connect better and more with the earth.

Sun Salutations

It also resembles the pose of a cobra serpent. Lie down with your stomach on the ground. Using your palm hands, lift your upper part of your body (from the waist upwards while still lying down) face up to the sun. Inhale and exhale slowly, and you will start feeling connected, feel more sense of power and heat building up from within your body. You can choose to either close or open your eyes.

Anjaneyasana

This pose involves stretching your quad and psoas muscles. Its connection with the chakras makes sense because it's associated with the fight-or-flight mechanism. It is also connected with the first or the root chakra. Inhale and exhale five breaths to allow more time for your muscles to transmute residual flight or fight energy into a calm yet courageous inner strength.

Warrior II

Just like the name, pose like a warrior with your hands stretched outside and one leg stretched and the other slightly bent. The pose helps you dig deeper into your determination and strength.

Bridge Pose

Lie flat on the ground and lift your body using your upper back and support your pose with the souls of the feet firmly against the ground. This pose will help stimulate your throat chakra and help your root chakra to release excess energy. You can also use this pose while trying to balance your sacral, solar plexus, and the heart chakras.

Wide-Legged Forward Fold

Stretch your legs and lower your head to touch the ground while also supporting yourself with your hands. This pose will open your lower back and groin muscles. This will give an opportunity to your root chakra to release energy into your body.

Savasana

Lie down while facing upwards to allow total support by the earth beneath your body. Inhale and exhale smoothly while repeating the words 'I am safe, I am supported' with every cycle of your breathing. When we approach life from a grounded perspective, we tend to be more calm and happy, and this pose provides an opportunity to do just that while making us stronger within ourselves.

Chapter 8: Chakra Massages

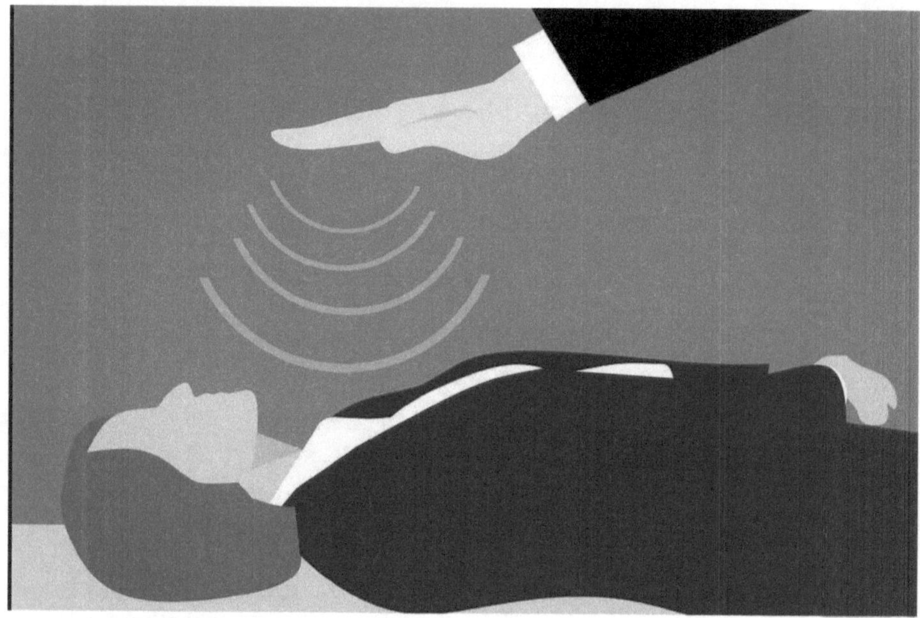

There are various massage techniques that people can use to improve their focus and connect with their chakras. There are several massage techniques you can try, such as:

Deep-Tissue Massage

Practicing this form of massage on your back is the first step you should take. The deep-tissue practice is not necessarily deep but rather slow and specific to a particular part. The main goal is to massage a particular muscle in a focused and slow manner using a broadening stroke or lengthening stroke meaning with or across the fiber, respectively.

When performing deep-tissue massage, the biggest advantage is focusing on the fascia or connective tissue. According to research, the connective tissue is the wiring of the energy flow in the human body. The fascia, on the other hand, acts as the conduit through which the energy in our body flows. This will enable us to focus on the erector spinae muscles with the determination to work with prana or chakra energy.

Practice lengthening strokes on your iliocostalis, longissimus, and the spinalis. Also, practice broadening strokes on the gluteus media, which will enable you to open the flow of the energy that connects prana with the legs. Also, practice broadening stroke on the longissimus.

Reflexology

Another technique is the "chakra" foot reflexology massage. The reflexology practice focuses on two chakra aspects: Chakra's physical location and the endocrine gland that is associated with each chakra either through close proximity or related function. The physical locations are situated along with the head reflex points on your feet and along the spinal as well.

The root chakra is located at the sacrum, and the root chakra reflex in your foot is in the sacral reflex on your foot. The seventh chakra reflex is found on the big toe's distal portion. The chakras are associated with the main endocrine glands.

All the other chakras are positioned in the feet as well. Also, there are other places that connect to the chakras such as sciatic nerve which connect with the root chakra, uterus connects to the sacral chakra, and the solar plexus and heart reflex connect to the third chakra and fourth chakra respectively.

Energy Work

Another technique is the chakra energy work. The light touch is the focus of the energy work over chakra while also focusing on the intended purpose. Focus on the connection and intention as well. Focus your visualization on two aspects, including working with the right (visual, intuitive) and left (analytic, logical) sides of your brain. Visualize colored energy in a spinning wheel on each part of the chakra (on the right brain).

Life Energy Massage

It is one of the most popular techniques. The main focus of life energy massage session is the advanced healing energy to clear the body. The cleansing involves getting rid of old feelings or habitual thought patterns. The session will enable you to clear negative thinking, clear past traumas, expansive feelings, improved sleep, increase energy, etc.

It's a gentle hand-on kind of session.

Chakra Foot Massage

In this form of chakra massage therapy, start by preparing a tub, foot bath, a small basin or a large bowl here bot your feet can fit comfortably. Lay a towel beside you to set and dry your legs and protect your floor. Add several teaspoons of sea or Epsom salt (you can also use coarse sea salt which is readily available in many grocery stores). Fill the very hot water, but it should not be too hot to hurt burn your legs. You can wait for the water to get cold for a few minutes.

You can also add few drops of recommended essential oil and an oil blend, perform massage on both feet, one at a time. When you are done with massaging one foot, put it in water as you massage the second one. After massaging both feet, place them in water and let them stay there for 10 to 15 minutes as long as the water is still hot. That's why it is still important to prepare very hot water. Breathe in and exhale smoothly. You can perform this form of meditation while listening to cool music; the use of chakra affirmations is also great. You can also prepare an inspiring statement that you can be reading while practicing this meditation.

For instance, if you are practicing root chakra, you can say, "I am grounded, I am safe, and the process of life is trustworthy."

You can also use the color that represents the chakra you are trying to heal. For your root chakra, use a red towel or blanket and so on for the rest of the chakras.

The main difference between getting a chakra massage and other types of massages like the regular massage is the knowledge about the chakra locations by chakra professionals massage providers. The expert giving you chakra massages will be able to facilitate your body's connection with your wisdom. They will be able to connect with you as a client or their patient properly, their main focus will be to balance or heal your chakra, they will be able to align the healing process with your intentions for concrete solutions. They will prepare the room and make sure it's warm and has a receptive environment to enable the quality meditation process and effective healing.

How Different Chakras Can Be Healed or Balanced Through Massage Therapy

Root chakra: With this chakra regarded as the foundation of the whole chakra system, it's good health is required just like the rest of the chakras. A professional chakra massage therapist will recommend the stimulation of your back through reflexology and balancing massage.

Solar Plexus: Located above the navel and below the heart, it is also regarded as the power center. Our power center can experience imbalance in situations such as the transition from adolescence to adulthood, dealing with a job loss or transition of your career. A professional chakra therapist will recommend deep-tissue massage in your back to realign the chakras.

Throat Chakra: This chakra is represented in throat and neck areas. A chakra massage expert will not just master the massage practice and perform it on you but will also master the communication practice as well. They will help with massaging your neck and throat areas to help you have a relaxing and comfortable expression and communication.

Crown Chakra: This is a chakra that helps connect with the higher purpose and relate to your wisdom. When this chakra is in good condition, you will are able to enjoy the full joy of our universe and feel blissful. The use of aromatherapy and deep-tissue massage will greatly in giving you this desirable feeling.

Use of Clockwise Circular Stroke

You can also practice this form of massage using water medicated and soluble oils alongside with the herbs. The root chakra can be massaged on the coccyx using dashmoola oil, which is formed from a blend of 10 herbs. The sacral chakra regulates creativity, sexual functions, and water balance. Dilute essential oil used for sacral chakra and massage the sacrum or the lower abdomen. For solar plexus, massage the navel area with ginger oils and peppermint.

The heart chakra is massaged at the upper back and the center of the chest using diluted basil oil. The throat chakra is massaged on the throat using oil that is infused with calamus. The third eye can be massaged with triphala or oil infused with a rose at the center of your forehead. The crown chakra is massaged at its chakra point as well, which is at the top of the head.

Massage therapies are excellent solution when looking for a way to balance and heal your chakras. In most cases, when one chakra is not allowing energy to flow freely either because of imbalance or blockage, massages will be of great help. Massages are applied to the correct places and will help you restore their correct energy. It is also easy to correct your chakra, especially if you are new and trying to heal or balance the chakra because you will identify with exact chakra points and master their locations. It is also advisable for you to combine massages with other practices such as health and the right diet, exercise, and meditation.

When there is a smooth flow of energies through your chakras, you will have stable and balanced mental, physical, emotional, and spiritual health. Chakra massage therapy is an excellent technique which does not only help you realign your chakras but also make you feel better, relax, and rejuvenated after the chakra massage sessions.

Chapter 9: Chakras and Auras

Auras are bio-magnetic fields of energies that surround us and are our energy blueprint. It can extend from several feet to a few inches.

Auras just like chakras can also be seen during meditations, with the inner eye, with psychic perception or healing sessions. Both aura and chakra can also be seen with the naked eye after more focus, training, meditation, and learning the knowledge of the human energy field. There are also those people who can see chakra or aura without training. There are also those who take time before been able to get spiritual power to view aura even after years of training.

Auras, just like chakras, can be separated into several other elements. It is easy to know the moods of certain people if you have an idea of what color to relate to their moods without even reading or examining their minds.

Auras enable you to observe the energy of love merging between two couples in love. Two arguing friends will have their energy focused on energy and their auras get thinner. There are several auric or energy fields which make up the auras which include:

Physical Field – Human beings can observe without training and changes based on your health and well-being.

Etheric Field – Changes based on the flow of energy and handles the exchange of energy between the physical body and universal energy.

Emotional Field – Affected by tension and stress

Mental Field – Changes depending on your focus or confusion. it is around your crown head

The Astral Field – Is the energy field is existing on its own plane free from confines of space and time. The work is done on all chakras to heal and perform their functions appropriately benefit the astral field.

The Etheric Template Field – It is responsible for representing our physical being in the spirit plane

The Celestial Field – Represents the etheric field as a template in the physical plane. It's super energetic and has access to all the energies offered by the universe.

Casual Field – Has everything to do with the outcome of your life's direction. It is similar to the mental field, but it works on a spiritual plane. It directs our existence in the lower levels based on the universe with no confines of time and space.

There is also a belief that young children have extra-sensory perceptions which enable them to see auric layers and chakras. However, they later shut down these unique powers after adults tell them they see something that does not exist. The children experience these powerful techniques because of the need to connect more with the environment they perceive does not support their involvement or with their physical existence.

Chakra and aura are connected very deeply since the aura produces out the information into the world where your chakras. Your root chakra makes you feel safe and grounded, and this will be projected out in the aura. On the other hand, if your solar plexus feel insecure and weak, you will project this feeling to the world. The aura is a blend of all the information your chakras send out and when your spiritual connection, emotional health and mood change, your colors change as well. However, for chakra's color, they remain constant and are deeply anchored. The color of the chakra can only change if a major event occurs.

Both chakras and auras constitute the individual's spiritual colors. They are also important to the health of a human being. The two channels of energy can also get blocked when the individual is suffering from illness or stress and affect the general health of a person. Specific forms of yoga, meditations, Reiki, and other scientific methods are practiced to purify auras and open blocked chakras to restore good health and the general well-being. The thickness, size, and shape of the chakras and auras describe many things about an individual. The more powerful and strong the aura is, the more fascinating the person, the clear (spacious-thickness-openness) your chakra, the healthier and stronger the person.

Both auras and chakras are capable of revealing a particular disease affecting an individual. When both chakras and auras are weak, it becomes hard to deal with present life situations unless the energies are treated.

Chapter 10: Basic Chakra Exercises for Balance and Health

There are several exercises and their concepts that can significantly boost your chakras' balancing or ability to perform their functions or heal as well. Below are some of the exercises you can practice to balance your chakras:

Exercise 1: Getting Rid of Bad Energy

Stand or site with your back straight and enhance your balance by stretching your legs apart. Slightly bend your knees and allow your weight to lie in your pelvis. Relax and equally distribute the weight down your legs. You can either close your eyes or leave them open. Breathe in for a little time, and make sure you are fully relaxed while inhaling. With one quick thought, send a golden root deep down the earth from your feet souls. Send the second root from your spine to enable you to sit on your golden root's tripod.

Discharge and get rid of any thoughts, feelings, or other things that you don't want from your being and chakras. Don't mind about where you are dumping your unwanted things from your being because the earth can handle anything through recycling or neutralization.

Draw up the energy from the earth, hold it, cherish it as it passes along all the roots, you will notice you are feeling stronger like a tree with roots firmly entrenched in its base. You are free to practice this exercise as long as you like.

When you feel strong and cleansed, slightly withdraw your roots but always know that you are in constant contact and intimate with the earth through your root chakra through your feet's souls. Therefore, It is important to ensure that your root chakra is always open.

Exercise 2: Filing Youself With Empowered Energy

To effectively practice this exercise, start by performing Exercise 1 that we have just discussed. This will help you to perform this second one with ease.

Lift your hands to face the sky and draw the energy from the sun from both the crown of your head and your palms. Allow the stream of silver energy to flow in and feel it as it passes through your heart and mix with the energy from the universe.

Aloud or silently, give thanks for all the things that have come your way. Feel the energy ""prana"" and its strength from both the sky and the earth, this is the moment when your spiritual energies also mingle with your earthly energy and power. It is also the excellent bonding of your human self and your soul. Feel energized, powerful, strength, renewed, and refreshed. You will also feel whole, and it's important to note and be aware of your immense potential.

When you feel ready, put your hands down and cup them around your heart while saying thankful words for the things that have happened in your life or situations. While still holding energies from both the sky and earth, gently withdraw your feet souls from the earth, which also translates to withdrawing your root chakra from the universe. Always ensure you stay in contact with the universe to keep your root chakra open.

Exercise 3: Protection Exercise

This exercise is purposely meant to protect yourself, especially if you feel you are surrounded by the toxic environment or you feel you are around someone or people who drain your "good energies."

Inhale and stay relaxed as much as possible. Form an imagination in your mind about a glamorous white flower at your head crown with wide-opened petals. Allow the white flower to close tightly and drop your focus to your brow with another flower, which is now blue in color and allow it to close tightly together with the petals as well. Move on to the next part and allow your thoughts to focus on your throat with its sky blue flower with opened petals, which also closes as well. Next, focus on your heart with a beautiful green flower and allow it to close tightly.

Also, allow the yellow flower and orange flower to close tightly in your solar plexus and sacral chakra respectively. Lift your arms and cross them across your chest. Slightly bow your head down and imagine a midnight blue cloak next to you and allow it to wrap around you to protect you from these external distractors that can negatively affect your chakras.

- Strike a Pose (Dance)

This is a form of simple dance that you think enables you to calm your nerves. This time you will dance it with all the seven chakras in your mind. Allow the rhythm to guide you and move your body freely to dispel any negative thoughts or feelings. Open, heal, and balance your root chakra. Combine this chakra with other forms of chakra exercises.

- Mindful Walking

Whether you are walking down in a crowded town or city or you are having a nature walk. Have awareness as you take each step. Focus on your breathing as well. Feel your feet as they touch the ground and note the sensation with every touch. These will help you balance your root chakra. Also, perform this exercise in combination with other chakra exercises to fully balance your root chakra.

- Get Moving

Root chakra is quite convenient because even moving around or performing simple house chores is one process of healing your root chakra. The key is to feel sensation during your movement and create awareness in your body. Awareness is always emphasized in chakras because they are vital for healing.

- Take a Bath or Shower

Rinse yourself off or take a bath. Create awareness while taking a shower and be aware of yourself and your body as you shower. This will enable you to heal and balance your root chakra.

A Summary of Helpful Exercises and Practices to Heal The Chakras

Root Culture: Grounding yourself to the earth will be helpful, and that includes walking barefoot on grass, sand, and soil. Practice strong and grounded yoga poses like mountains and trees. Reinstate the roots by learning how to forgive transgressions and mistakes committed to you, whether in your adults life or childhood life. Also, learn to provide things that impart basic needs, security, and safety on a day-to-day basis.

Sacral Chakra: Listening to what your body says, self-affirmation. Practice yoga for balance, swimming, walking, slow hikes, destiny manifestation, intimate touch, and dreams.

Solar Plexus: Practicing gentle exercises, belly breath work like yoga twists, Lion's breathe meditation, and practicing the release of stomach muscles.

Heart Chakra: Practice deep breathing to have cleared lungs and while your shoulders are drawn back and down for your heart to open. Stretch your body and practice chest opening exercises. Stimulate your limbic system through exercises such as rebounding. Other exercises for the heart chakra include hikes, swimming, shoulder, slow and long walks, warm baths, and chest and shoulder massage.

Throat Chakra: Perform deep breathe (make sure it's diaphragmatic), meditate, get words or issues out of your chest, speak with brevity and truthfully, stay near or inside the water, walking under the big sky and inhale in the fresh air. Practice visualization while speaking the truth to your colleague, friend, or family. Practice regularly on how to produce sounds that resemble those of the soothing winds.

The Third-Eye Chakra: Learn to practice Long stretches, yoga, and meditation, simple and repetitive exercises like swimming, hiking, or even "Tai Chi" if you are a fan. Try to put or get a greater picture into perspective by opening up your mind and involving yourself in adventure activities like visiting magnificent landscapes.

Crown Chakra: Think positively, meditate. Learn to be aware of when breathing. Practice other forms of exercises that heal or balance other chakras to enhance

Chapter 11: Astrology of the Chakra

Astrology and chakra complement each other, and this is interesting because astrology major concern is the outer world while chakra involves the inner world. Learning about their connection also enhances our understanding of these two psychological systems.

When we look at the chakras in more deeply, we will learn that most of them possess at least three diverse aspects, including spiritual (balanced), masculine (extroverted) and feminine (introverted). In other words, chakras can be experienced at the center of the spine in a well-balanced manner or to its left or right side. When the chakras are on their left or right side, there are associated with 12 Zodiac (zodiac astrological) signs.

Each chakra's psychological energy is manifested in various unique ways. For instance, if you experience your chakra in its extra masculine mode (Gemini), the throat or fifth chakra will manifest to the physical outer world through interpersonal communications. However, the feminine side or Virgo will manifest itself through the internal thought process. Throat chakra controls the mystical mind or mentality aspect that communicates with the spirit.

Cornelius Agrippa, a traditional esoteric source, expresses in the following ay using the same idea: Saturn rules Capricorn and Aquarius by night and day respectively. Jupiter rules Pisces and Sagittarius by night and day respectively, and Mars rules Scorpio and Aries by night and day respectively, Venus rules by Taurus and Libra by night and day respectively, Mercury rules Virgo and Gemini by night and day respectively. The Moon and Sun rule one sign each, Cancer and Leo, respectively. Chakras manifest in their centers of energies in a spiritually-balanced manner surpassing the dualistic qualities of the zodiacal wheel.

The twelve Zodiac signs are directly related to the seven chakras. You can simply spin the Zodiac to enable them to fall into place or in line with the placements of the chakras.

The three outer planets also fall into line with the root, sacral and solar plexus which are the first three chakras. Based on zodiacal signs, they are normally associated with control or rulership. The root chakra is ruled by Saturn, the sacral chakra is ruled by Jupiter, Solar Plexus is ruled by Jupiter, Heart Chakra is ruled by Venus. The throat chakra is ruled by Mercury, and the Third eye is ruled by Sun and Moon while the crown is the only chakra with no planetary association. Crown chakra is said to beyond any karma and therefore is not possible to compare it with any planet.

In yoga philosophy, each chakra center represents a sort of memory zone or "storage space" for life impressions and karmas. Everything we experience, think, and feel is packed into the spinal column in the form of energy fields. This is the reason why we are able to pick up the habitual behaviors which are built over time and engraved into our subconscious psyche and retrieved on a regular basis when we want pick up the habit again.

The Scientific Relationship Between Chakra Personality and Astrological Signs

Each personality consists of basic elements of the Chakra system even though in varying combinations. Depending on the existing patterns of the chakra functioning in an individual, subtle energies will focus themselves in various areas of the chakra system and then deployed to heal or balance the chakra parts. Although each person's center of energies will experience a varying degree of functionality, everyone has a specific chakra that is dominant than the others. For instance, if you are the intellectual type, your dominant chakra might be the throat chakra while your artistic friends will have his heart chakra as his principal chakra. The dominant or principal chakra can also be regarded as chakras that are more emphasized in a personality.

Let's us use the subpersonality model as your basis for utilizing the corresponding system. Each chakra has its own personifications or traits.

Chakras can also be described in the following way: The root chakra or Saturn can be called "inner architect" or "inner politician" in a metaphorical sense. The sacral chakra or Jupiter can be known as "inner optimist" or "inner preacher," the solar plexus or Mars can be known as "inner warrior," The heart chakra or Venus can be referred to as "inner lover" or "inner artists," the throat chakra or Mercury is the "inner thinker" or "inner communicator." The third eye or the lunar is also known as the "inner queen" or "inner mother." The crown chakra or solar is also known as the "inner king" or "inner father."

Chakra Interpretation Using Signs

We have learned from our previous discussions earlier in this chapter on how the chakras closely correspond to the twelve signs; you just need to spin your Zodiac until you are sure that you Leo and Cancer are placed at the top of the wheel. To know the dominant chakra or the one with more emphasis, you will need to get clues by looking at how the planets in a person are placed within the various existing signs. For instance, if Libra or Taurus have a large constellation of planets, your dominant chakra is more likely to be the heart chakra, while the large constellation of planets in

Aries or Scorpio would indicate the focus is on the solar plexus and so on.

Each planet's amplification in a certain chakra level is different from one another. For instance, when Jupiter and Saturn are located in one specific chakra level at different times, each one will have a different impact. Saturn is specifically placed on chakra centers that experience frustrations, growing challenges, or denial. Also, Saturn placement may indicate the level at which your greatest depth of wisdom exists. Such wisdom comes from you're the past generations or lives. If Saturn is placed on your certain chakra, you will have to work extra harder to achieve your goal in that Saturn-inhabited chakra center.

The rewards for Saturn inhabited chakra center is always expected to be greater if you work hard on them. On the other hand, Jupiter placement on a specific chakra indicates that you will get good fortune or blessings on that chakra. Jupiter-inhabited chakra has more or excess life energies expressions and fluidity in their openings.

Moon, sun and ascendant are also another very important area to learn and understand the chakras focus on your life. Sun in Gemini suggests an intensified focus upon your throat chakra of expression through communication as well as the attention on mentality. Sun in Capricorn would direct the focus on the earth plane and success establishment, balance, and recognition. In astrology, the Moon, Sun, and Ascendant are primary indicators that have specific shades of meaning each, and they have been among the main topics of discussions by astrologers for years.

The moon is associated with the chakra with emotional challenges, while ascendant indicates the present personality in your current life in terms of the habitual ways of relating and thinking. The sun, on the other hand, indicates the chakra direction in which you desire to go and which one of them is trying to display creative manifestation.

Chapter 12: The Science Behind Chakras

Chakra is all about energy flow through Nadis (Sanskrit word for rivers, meaning they are vessels through which the energy flows through the chakra system in our being. Our body has many chakras, but we focus on seven chakras only, which starts at the base of the spine, follows the spine's curvature and ends at the crown head.

In science and specifically in Quantum Physics, "everything is energy." Many things and items around us are made up of atoms.

Atoms have other subatomic particles which are three in total, the electrons, neutrons, and protons. Electrons whizz around the atom's outer side while neutrons and protons are fixed together at the atom's center. The movement of electrons is so quick that we never know their exact location at any given moment.

It's human nature to think of matter as solid and space as empty. But in reality, we live in a world where there is no solid reality around us. Even though items like chairs are made up of atoms, in

reality, they are not solid static items.
Scientifically, we say at a subatomic level, atoms
are made up of 99.99% space.

Your body also consists of constantly moving and
changing the mass of energy. Everything around
you and in your being is a field of constantly
fluctuating energy.

Energetic bonds hold together all matter, which
consists of atoms, the majority of which is space.
Energy movement is important to life. When we
breathe, function, think, and even rest, electrical
energy flow via nerve pathways and neurons
through our bodies. Major chakras positions
correspond to the main nerve, ""bundles"" or
nerve plexus.

Metaphysical theories also state that every chakra
controls specific organs and has their own
frequency level as well. Looking at what each
chakra represents will help you understand these
metaphysical theories.

Root Chakra controls hips, lower back, and legs,
and is where the feelings of security and safety are
experienced. The sacral chakra, on the other hand,

presides over the kidneys and reproductive system and the feelings of sensuality, overall connection, and intimacy. Solar plexus reigns over the liver, pancreas, intestines and similar organs as well as self-esteem, temperament, and ego. Heart chakra controls the thymus region and heart region and governs our forgiveness, compassion, and love for oneself and others.

Throat chakra control thyroid glands, and it's where the individual's expression and communication ability and creativity are fostered. The third eye chakra presides over facials regions and pituitary gland and a person's reasoning and intuition. The crown chakra controls the amygdala and other parts of the brain and is responsible for controlling emotions, memory, spirituality, and aggression.

Many scientific studies have established that emotions and thoughts play a vital role in the physical health of a human being. Controlled and healthy breathing contributes to excellent brain function and complete health. Chakra practice also enables an individual to engage with purposeful and meaningful attributes of life. While there is no direct scientific link about how chakra helps people deal with their personal problems, the chakra practice has helped very many individuals recover from abuse, trauma, addiction, and other personality and emotional problem. Chakra helps people become healthier.

Chakra System and Biological Science

The nervous system consists of nerve tissues that are responsible for causing or enabling most of our energetic process to take place within our bodies. Our nervous system also controls the coordination of our involuntary and voluntary actions and transmits signals to the brain from different body parts.

The nervous system consists of two major parts. One part is the Central Nervous System (CNS) within the spinal cord and the brain. Peripheral Nervous system (PNS) is the other part that connects both the spinal cord and the brain with the rest of the body via Nadis "or 'river' like nerve fibers." PNS is what correlates with the chakras.

Within the PNS, there are nerve bundles of different categories, but the one considered most relevant is the PNS's Autonomic nervous system. It is responsible for controlling the automatic and involuntary responses of a human body. For instance, our sneezing, digestion, heart rate, breathing, and swallowing are regulated by the hypothalamus, which is the control center of most of the PNS's autonomic functions.

Autonomic Nervous System is then divided into the Parasympathetic Nervous System which is activated when digesting and resting and the Sympathetic Nervous System which is activated to move energy in the course of emergencies for the flight and fight responses.

The parasympathetic Nervous System is the part of the nervous system, which has huge relevance to the positions where chakras are located. Nerve bundles are also associated with our body's major glands, which are also vital for the functioning of our bodies through secreting hormones in our bloodstream. Vagus nerve is also responsible for the stimulation of our body hormones, which play a vital part in our body's chemistry.

Hormones and nerves send information between organs and cells and affect several aspects of different processes in our bodies. These processes include mood, growth, sexual development, brain functioning, digestive process of breaking down the food, sleeping, and managing stress. The aging process occurs partly because of a decrease in the production of hormones. Dimethyltryptamine or DMT is another hormone secreted in the brain by the pineal gland is associated with heightened creativity, causing extra experience out of our body as well as association with psychic abilities.

In a nutshell, all the chakras are associated with the main networks of the nerve system within your body which connect via the main Vagus nerve from the brain and spine to the glands responsible for the functioning of the body and hormone production.

The Vagus conveys sensory information regarding our body organs' state to the central nervous system. It goes down the body after leaving the brain and scatter around our internal organs. It also acts as a "reset" button where our automatic, internal alarm system is counteracted, resulting in "flight or fight" response. Stimulation of the Vagus might lead to positive health benefits especially because we live in a society where it is normal to have subconscious fear such as fear of money, stability, a job's status, and other things.

Numerous studies have been conducted and documented stating that stimulation of the Vagus nerve can help in dealing with several other illnesses such as depression (especially the type that is regarded as treatment-resistant) and specific forms of epilepsy.

The most effective method of Vagus nerve stimulation, which is also natural is the deep belly breathing (also called Pranayama in Indian during ancient times). Other methods of stimulation are meditation (chakra forms of meditation can greatly help) and exercise.

The ancient description for the energies present in our bodies was referred to us the Kundalini which stems from the spine at the base and winds its way to the top of the head. Kundalini is in most cases or according to ancient times compared to a serpent or a snake. To awaken Kundalini, you are required to perform deep meditation, a sense of bliss, and enlightenment. The Kundalini serpent is said to coil three times, and this corresponds with the Vagus functioning, which is said to connect to the spine exactly 3 times. Although ancient descriptions are still unclear in many ways, the metaphors used to relate to very accurate information on human well-being.

Chakra science appears to be an exploration of metaphysical phenomena's scientific validation. Quantum physics suggests observation affects matter and even collapses wave-function (possible state of the physical system which is represented mathematically) quantum physics finds the accurate state of a physical system through actual measurement and observation. The act of observation is what determines the materialization of a particular state. According to quantum physics, by placing our focus on our nadis and chakras, we are more likely to affect the energy flow and improve our well-being and sense of peace. They are especially important when you are intending to create real improvements and changes in your body.

Chakras are referred to us the energy powerhouses that draw energy or prana (universal life-force) into the body and are responsible for spinning. They distribute "prana" or "energy" to other areas of our bodies. Every chakra is responsible for influencing the functions of the body where it is located in the spine. Chakras are responsible for influencing the activities of vital glands in our bodies. Besides influencing the functions of the nervous system, they also feed in good bio-energies and interact with the lymphatic system and endocrine glands.

Most of what you see in the world today is a combination of energy and matter. Our existence as a human being is a combination of both the body and consciousness. Our body as a matter is in existence because of consciousness. Chakra practice proved many years ago that energy and matter co-exist for a body to have existence. Science proved just recently that energy and matter are indeed one and the same thing. Science has also proved that every cell in our body is embedded with intelligence. Every cell consists of chemicals with each one having energy and intelligence. It is this combination that forms a body-mind system.

In the chakra system, if the body is alive and present, then the particular energies for all the chakras are also present. The body is the basic, and if the body is dead, there is no energy, hence no activity present.

The energy mechanism of a person breaks when death happens, and so the body's sense of response mechanism also dies. When a person is alive, his body produces energy which can also be healed, replaced, or balanced. The mechanism of the body is made from many other different parts, including digestion, circulation, metabolism, respiration, urination, excretion, and other parts. When these parts are functioning as required, the body is then able to produce energy constantly. If one part suffers a major break down or upset, the entire mechanism is affected, and the body dies.

Just like science, every mechanism in your body is important. Chakras are created through all these parts of the human body. Chakra can also be said to be the byproduct of our body and the energies present.

We also keep the knowledge of chakras in mind, and if our mind was not functioning as required, then we don't know anything about them.

Each one of us has crucial energy in our body, and we spend a lot of our time dissipating these energies in different places. If you wish to achieve something or you are ambitious, you need to understand your energy more deeply. It will be easier and also possible to align your chakras and energy if you understand them better.

Science has also proved the existence of meridians in our bodies. According to science, we exist in a mental and spiritual universe as well as in energy fields where our reality is also created by our thoughts, emotions, and absolute love.

One study by a former medical school professor and author of "The Biology of Belief" is one of the groundbreaking works which have proved that signals coming from outside the human cells control our biology. It shows that if we retain our thinking, we can change our bodies with those particular thoughts at that moment.

Our hearts has electromagnet fields that are powerful rhythmically and can be detected by sensitive instruments several feet away. According to research, when we experience various emotions, our heart's field alters. When this is registered in our brains, it triggers certain effects that prompt the cells, DNA, and water studied in vitro to behave in a specific manner. There is also more growing evidence that suggests the heart's energetic interactions have the capability of underlying human consciousness' vital aspects and intuition. The study concludes that our bodies are energetic beings physically, spiritually, and in our minds and that our reality is created through our thoughts, actions, and emotions.

It also means that for us to explore and understand deeper into the science of energy existence and healing, we first need to understand that we do not just matter. The chakra system, just like science, states that for our body to exist, we are powered by good energies which enable us to have a healthy life. We also understand our existence and body-mind better if we explore and

study the science of energy and the deeper
meaning of our existence.

Chapter 13: Healing Your Chakras

The chakra system is a beneficial tool as a diagnostic tool. The signs of imbalance are shown by physical feelings of illnesses and tension in the position where the chakra center of energy lies. Knowing which chakra is problematic will enable you to identify the type of healing required to work on a particular chakra and heal your physical body, spirit, and mind.

Healing Chakra Exercises

There are various types of healing chakra exercises, they include:

- **Visualization**

This is a form of healing chakra exercise that involves channeling the power of your mind to enable you to create change that is positive. It also requires that you visualize while envisioning yourself insulated and protected in bright light. The light should balance perfectly with all chakras, this also means you go for the color that matches the chakra you wish to heal. You can also use white light, which is also perfect for all chakra and what most trainers will also recommend to you and also when you are not sure which color represent your chakra. More practice on your visualization will make you better and successful when healing your chakra.

- **White Sage**

A white sage is created by wafting the smoke from the burning white sage, which is completely dried. This will enable you to tune-up your energy in a quick fashion than other similar forms of exercises like taking a bath. The burning white sage smoking will look like incense. Catch the burning embers if possible and place it in a plate, dish, bowl, or any other convenient place and move it around yourself as if you are bathing. After the burning white sage healing exercise, extinguish it by either sealing it in an enclosed area like a mason jar or running it underwater.

- **Flower Essences**

A flower essence is either taken in water or under the tongue, and it's used as a powerful vibrational remedy which is capable of shifting positive energy. While flower essence might be used to serve similar purposes or similar to aromatherapy oils but in truth, they are very different. Unlike aromatherapy, a flower essence does not have a scent, and they are preserved in water or brandy as blossom's healing vibration. You can purchase them from the health food stores. A flower essence is used to heal any chakra when it has difficulty. They can also heal multiple chakras or all of them.

- **Aromatherapy**

They are used to create healthy impact on our body and mind. Applying aromatherapy essential oil will help you achieve the goal of healing your chakras. Some of the aromatherapy examples include Patchouli/Vetiver for your root chakra, Ylang Ylang for your sacral chakra and Tangerine for your solar plexus chakra. Others include Rose for the heart chakra, Clary Sage for your Throat Chakra, Peppermint for your third eye and Lavender for the crown chakra.

Healing for Calm and Serenity Exercise

It combines both the third eye healing and the crown healing, and its purpose is to tune you up into your future and divine and force you into the moment. It involves placing one hand on your crown head, put the fingers of your other hand over your third eye chakra (the location between your to eyes). Hold on that position, inhale deeply and exhale gently and through both your hands, you start feeling your pulse. Perform the exercise for at least 5 minutes or until you feel your chakra is fully healed.

- **Healing for Harmony: Applies on Crown Chakra**

This exercise helps you attain the general peace and sense of harmony. It is also used when a person allows a better opening on his chakra and want to cool down after a long stressful event or day. Also, begin by placing your hand on top of your crown head. Using the fingers from the other hand, touch your nose at the tip. Breathe deeply until there is a feeling of pule points in every part.

- **Healing for Communication: Applies to Throat Chakra**

It is common for people to lose words while communicating, unable to think clearly or make a wise decision at the right time. This throat healing exercise will help you energize your throat chakra and make it powerful again for you to have your voice back. You will also find that your stress levels are down if your throat chakra is powerful enough to make excellent expressions.

Start by practicing your voice like an artist or a singer would do while preparing for a performance. Warm by chanting the vocal cords as your 'ohm' or any other sound that you perceive as relaxing. Put your hand on your crown head at the top. Relax and wait until you feel a pulse. Inhale and exhale gently until you start feeling your stress level is going down or your chakras are fully healed. Visualize words like worries, fear, and stress also exiting with the other negative energies out of your body.

- **A Selenite Wand**

A selenite wand is an energy balancer or detoxifier just like a white sage except that it doesn't produce smoke alarms. Place it a foot away from your body and use it to healing your energy by brushing it while paying special focus on the chakra part that you wish to heal. Place selenite in bright sunlight to cleanse it after using it.

Affirmations

Other tools that are considered powerful in chakra healing are the affirmations; these are positive statements that have the effect of healing and strengthening the misaligned parts of our being. When using affirmations, we are able to maintain focus on different facets of our life, one by one. Below are some of the examples of affirmations:

- Root Chakra – "I am filled with humbleness. I am enough as I am."
- Sacral Chakra – "I am strong, beautiful/handsome, radiant, and enjoy a passionate and healthy life."
- Solar Plexus – "I accept who I am. I accept that I have power, and I also accept I have weaknesses".

- The Heart Chakra – "Love answers everything in life; I am the giver and recipient of unconditional love."
- The Throat Chakra – "I am filled with positive thoughts, and I always communicate and express myself clearly and truthfully."
- The Third Eye Chakra – "I am a wise person, and I truly understand the meaning of life situations."
- The Crown Chakra – "I am full and filled with divine energy"

If you practice these affirmations statements for some period while healing your chakras, you will start seeing positive results.

Health Through Music

Each chakra has a sound healing frequency that it responds to and one of the famous techniques is the Solfeggio, which contains music frequencies that are used to make healing tones or sounds. Isochronic Chakra Suite is another common type of music used, and it consists of brainwave techniques for entertainment, including Tibetan singing bowl which is done in combination with Solfeggio frequencies.

Color Vibration

Another simple chakra healing exercise is practicing color vibration technique. We can heal our chakras by exposing ourselves to different color types representing the chakras. We can expose ourselves to various colors in our house, including our clothes, flowers, and the food that we prepare and eat to re-align and heal our chakras. Wearing color glasses can also help in absorbing the color vibrations that are required in our bodies.

Professional Energy Healers

Another way to help you with the healing of the chakras is by visiting a professional and experienced energy healer. The professionals will examine the energy levels of their clients and figure out the reason for experiencing an energy blockage.

The healer will then have the ability to provide advice on the most appropriate treatment options for healing a particular chakra and how to apply them as required. There are those professional healers who might give you chakra healing lessons or offer their clients, the chakra practices healing sessions. With the true professional healer, you will overcome any form of spiritual blockage that you might be experiencing.

Fire Breathing Technique

1. This is one of the most rejuvenating and relaxing healing techniques. Huge emotions might pass through you, and you might discover that you were unknowingly holding some of them. You are free to express anger and release tears so that you can heal completely and release all negative energies inside your body, mind, and soul. You can either choose to do it alone or with your partner as well.

2. Start by dropping any expectations and put your energy and mindset in a state of desire. Relax your mind and avoid too many thoughts on expectation or attachment.

3. Lie while facing up while your back is in the ground. Allow your jaw to relax and inhale

and exhale using your nose and mouth, respectively.

4. Feel as your belly is filling up and level your lower back against the ground as you exhale. You should feel tender rocking in the pelvis while performing this part.

5. While exhaling, squeeze your Kegels.

6. As you inhale, think about it and let the energy pull from your perineum in the first chakra as it follows your thoughts. You don't have to strain while pulling in the energy because you just need to use your thoughts and feel.

7. Inhale the energy and then exhale in this manner, every time you inhale in your root chakra, allow it to move on to the sacral chakra and then in your imaginations, form an energy cycle that will rotate from the root to sacral chakra. Then from the sacral chakra to solar plexus and then from solar plexus to heart and then from the heart to the third eye. From the third eye form another energy circle that will rotate to the

throat chakra and then from throat chakra to the crown head.

8. According to experts in this form of healing exercise, you are allowed to enlarge these energy circles and jump to one or two chakras. Say form an energy circle from the root chakra and up to the solar plexus or from solar plexus up to the third eye. All these enlarging or contracting the energy balls are done to heal the damaged chakra.

9. Keep breathing as you move energy circles and physically and gently moving your hips. This will give you space to pass through the whole process of rejuvenating your body energy and healing your chakra.

Balance Your Chakras with Acupuncture and Essential Oils

Chakra acupuncture involves the stimulation of spaces and points through the method acupuncture to balance the chakras and increase the flow of energy or prana. Acupuncture is the use of thin needles where they are inserted into a particular part of the body for a specific form of healing purposes. It is particularly famous in traditional Chinese forms of medicine and healing, but it's also applied to Indian's form of healing processes like chakra. For chakra acupuncture, it is the position of the chakra parts in your body that will complement this technique.

Using the chakra acupuncture technique, you will need to start with the crown head, followed by the root and heart chakra simultaneously. The needles will be safely inserted carefully in a particular part of your bodies, and if it's the crown, they will be inserted on the head. Don't worry, it's safe, and you will not have to worry about injuring your body because the thin needles will not go past the first layer of your skin.

It is important to pay fully focus on the chakra that you are treating one by one. The process will begin by the opening of the chakras. You will feel the energy flowing gently through your chakras. Breathing and focusing on your chakra deeply will help you open the chakras and intensify the flow of the energy through your body, mind, and soul. Acupuncture treatment of the chakras requires you to combine with the awareness to enable the treatment to be more efficient.

Essential Oils for Balancing Chakras

Essential oils are tools that have been time-tested and proved in the chakra healing practice. They are available for all types of ailments. Using other forms of healing while applying essential oil is an excellent choice to enhance the healing of chakra and promote the balancing of the chakras. Essential oils have a simultaneous effect on your spirit, mind, and body.

The essential oils have the ability to energize the underactive chakras and harness the overactive chakras to the required levels.

- **Sandalwood Oil For Root Chakra**

The Sandalwood oil is made from the sandalwood trees, heartwood, which is part of the sandalwood trees is steam distilled to make sandalwood oil. In Eastern cultures, sandalwood oil is considered as one of the sacred symbols. It is rich in anti-anxiety, calming, antidepressant properties and sedative.

Sandalwood oil can harmonize your emotions, calm your nervous system, provides you with a sense of stability and security. It is an excellent option if you are looking for a way to maintain or retain the issues or good energies of your root chakra.

Other examples of essential oil you can use for root chakra balancing include Back Pepper, Nutmeg, Cypress, Sweet Marjoram, Vetiver, Myrrh, and Patchouli.

- **Ylang Ylang Oil for Sacral Chakra**

The source of Ylang Ylang essential oil is the fragrant flowers of the tropical trees of the Cananga odorata species. The tree is from Indonesia. It as flowery and mild scent and it makes it well aphrodisiac aid and romantic.

Ylang Ylang is very helpful in helping in the calming of the agitation and fear of the sacral chakra when it is in its overactive form. The sedative oil has a tendency to heighten your sexual pleasure and boot the energies of your reproductive system. It is also required to be diluted it any available carrier oil before application. You can apply Ylang Ylang on your back while you are getting your massage at the lower back area.

Other examples of the essential oils for the fourth or sacral chakra include Neroli, Geranium, Lavender, Jasmine, Clary Sage and Mandarin.

- **Cinnamon essential Oil For Solar Plexus Chakra**

Cinnamon oil is fragrant and spicy, and it comes from aromatic Indian Spice Cinnamon. It has the capability of powering up and boosting your adrenal glands and gives you the power to attain positive self-confidence in anything you pursue or try to achieve or overcome.

Cinnamon has antidepressants and tranquilizing effects which enable it to relieve doubts, stress, fear, and confusion. Applying gentle oil massage on your stomach also has the capability of activating your third or solar plexus chakra.

Other examples of essential oils that can be applied to balance solar plexus chakra include Thyme, Peppermint (for calming overactive chakra), Chamomile Roman, Eucalyptus, Lemon, Bergamot and Juniper
Berry.

- **Rose Oil For Heart Chakra**

Floral and sweet fragrant Rose oil is extracted and distilled form it's flower's petals. Rose oil is also therapeutic and is capable of managing hormonal issues, menstrual, and skin disorders in women. It is considered as an aphrodisiac essential oil, and it's also capable of boosting your romantic life.

It helps reduce trauma, insomnia, depressions, anxiety, and stress. As the emotional hub, the heart makes the rose essential oil has the perfect oil for anointing and balancing or aligning the root chakra. Massage the breastbone using 2-3 drops of the rose essential oil and the massage should also include the body's back area.

Other examples of essential oils for the Heart Chakra include Grapefruit, Lavender (for calming the chakra), Bergamot Neroli, Clary Sage, Sweet Marjoram, Melissa and Cypress.

- **Eucalyptus Oil For Throat Chakra**

It comes from the Eucalyptus tree itself in its evergreen nature, and the leaves and twigs are picked and steam distilled to make Eucalyptus oi. The oil has several properties, including antibacterial characteristics and woody aromas. These properties make it perfect to be used for all issues or problems affecting the respiratory system, such as flu, cold, sore throat, cough, congestions, etc.

The Eucalyptus oil has properties such as stimulating effect, and it's used to stimulate the human mind and get rid of lethargy and heaviness. Using two to three drop of the Eucalyptus, you can boost the regulation of your throat chakra and help clear your throat and airways

Other types of essential oils you can use to balance your Heart Chakra: Peppermint, Lemon, Basil, Roman chamomile, Spearmint, and Coriander.

Lavender Essential Oil For Third Eye Chakra

Its source is the aromatic Lavender flowers. It is a famous essential oil that is useful in aligning or balancing all the seven chakras. You can massage using a moderate mixture of carrier oil with about three drops of Lavender oil on your third eye position, which is the location between your eyes. The properties of Lavender oil include energy rejuvenation and relaxation when inhaled.

Other examples of essential oils that can be used to balance your third eye include Lemon, Frankincense, Juniper, Rosemary, and Sandalwood.

Frankincense Oil For Crown Chakra

It is considered as sacred oil. It is widely used for anointing purposes in Middle Eastern cultures. Its source is oleoresin from the Frankincense tree. It has a sweet aroma with properties such as sedative and antidepressants. These characteristics can help you soothe both your body and mind.

You are required to diffuse about 6 to 8 drops of the Frankincense essential oil just above the crown head to enable you to regulate and balance your seventh or crown chakra.

Other examples of the crown chakra include Neroli, Geranium, Rose, Myrrh, and Lavender.

- **Crystal for Chakras Balance**

Crystals can also be used to balance the chakras on your body. You are either supposed to place them on a particular part of the body, carry or wear them. Your needs are the determinant of the frequency that you require for balancing. Focus on your symptoms to get to know the right moment to balance your chakras. There is a specific crystal for a particular chakra that you will need to use. The crystals used for the healing of the chakras have various attributes or properties, including their color, personal or intuitive resonance, and energetic quality.

List of Chakra Crystal

Each chakra is associated with one or several other crystals. Depending on the energy center you wish to focus on, below is a list of healing crystal and the chakra that they are capable of healing.

- Root Chakra crystals: Fire Agate, Tiger's Eye, Black Tourmaline, Hematite, Bloodstone
- Sacral chakra crystals: Carnelian, Coral, Moonstone, Citrine
- Solar Plexus Chakra crystals: Calcite, Topaz, Malachite, Citrine
- Heart Chakra crystals: Jade, Rose Quartz, Green Tourmaline, Green Calcite\
- Throat chakra crystals: Turquoise, Lapis Lazuli, Aquamarine

- Third Eye Chakra crystal: Black Obsidian, Amethyst, Purple Fluorite
- Crown Chakra crystal: Amethyst, Selenite, Diamond, Clear Quartz

Below is a brief summary of the above-listed crystals that are used for healing.

- Agate
  - Helps in staying grounded
  - Aligns the human physical body with the etheric body
  - Responsible for stimulating the root chakra
  - Boost the positive condition of the sexual and bowel organs
  - Intensifies emotions and passion
- Amethyst
  - Helps in clearing the mind
  - Helps in getting rid of addictive behaviors
  - Facilitates meditation
  - Helps know the root cause of unbalanced chakra or illness
  - Helps you to know the patterns of self-destructive egos.

- - o Helps you feel native to planet earth
  - o Helps people to guide their communication
- Citrine
  - o Helps to clear thoughts
  - o Enhances energy and the physical stamina
  - o Enhances proper metabolism and endocrine system
  - o Helps overcome adversity and difficulty
  - o Magnifies manifestation and will power
  - o Enhances creativity
  - o Enables people to open their divine of energy
- Carnelian
  - o Helps one in taking action
  - o Builds courage, power, confidence, and passion
  - o Helps in detoxification and body purification from bad addictive habits like drug abuse and alcohol

- o Enables you to overcome anxiety when planning to take action
- Calcite (Orange Calcite)
  - o Helps in overcoming social phobias and shyness
  - o Helps in overcoming depression
  - o Enhances the functions of hormonal balances and endocrine system
  - o Helps in bringing energy field to the human body
- Diamond
  - o Promote vision and truth
  - o Helps in clearing the energy field
  - o Helps in clearing emotional body by getting rid of density in it
  - o Assists in connecting with domains of the higher level
  - o Used in supporting other crystals
- Fluorite
  - o Strengthens the teeth and bones
  - o Helps with vertigo and dizziness problem
  - o Enhances the balancing of the chemistry of the brain

- o Bring focus and structure to energies that are incoherent
  - o Help thinking clearly
  - o Can remedy dishonesty, instability, and confusion
  - o Clear cluttered thoughts and confusion
- Jade
  - o Balances and harmonizes the heart chakra
  - o Aids in physical and emotional well-being
  - o Attracts prosperity and abundance
  - o Strengthens the system of your energy distribution
- Lapis Lazuli
  - o Help in connecting with earthly gods
  - o Assist in discovering the nature of your inner divine
  - o Enhances divine inspiration
  - o Helps in clearing the body's energy system
  - o Assist in activating the third eye's psychic centers

- Moonstone
    - Enhances intuition
    - Promote clairvoyance
    - Helps in attuning a person to the energy of the moon
    - Assist in stabilizing female cycles
    - Assist in categorization personal emotions
    - Enables one to take appropriate action and be patience
    - Used in regressing past life and in meditation
- Obsidian (Black Obsidian)
    - Helps in grounding
    - Helps in clearing the auric field
    - Helps in getting rid of negative energies
    - Helps in getting rid of blockages and obstructions in the meridian system
- Quartz (Clear Quartz)
    - Helps in opening chakras
    - Helps in heightening awareness spiritually
    - Is programmable and has memory

- o Expands consciousness
  - o Amplifies the person's psychic abilities
  - o Encourages clarity
  - o Helps in stimulating the nervous system
  - o Enhances the growth of fingernails and hair
  - o Amplifies energy
- Rose Quartz
  - o Assist in healing the heart
  - o Helps in calming the mind
  - o Dispels suspicion and fear
  - o Reawakens trust
  - o Releases stress and tension
  - o Assist in releasing anxiety, worries, emotional traumas as a result of the past tragedies and the fear
  - o Assist in balancing the heart chakra

- Tiger's Eye
  - o Stimulates sex, solar plexus, and roots chakras
  - o Support vitality

- o Helps in strengthening the endocrine system
  - o Sharpens logic and activates intellectual and wise thinking and actions
  - o Helps in taking effective action
  - o Helps in energizing the body
- Tourmaline (Black Tourmaline)
  - o Clears the auric field
  - o Support the clearing of the heavy metals
  - o Helps in controlling and regulating energetic and electrical systems of the human body
  - o Helps in enhancing psychic protection
  - o Helps in untying oneself from addictive bad behaviors
- Turquoise
  - o Assist in increasing wealth
  - o Helps in increasing prana
  - o Helps in enhancing oxygen availability in our circulation systems

- o Assist in heightening the intelligence of human emotions
- o Assist in balancing the moods of a human being
- o Promotes self-acceptance, self-forgiveness, and release of regrets
- o Assist in protecting oneself from evil
- o Helps in stimulating the throat chakra

Have a Healthy Sex Life

It is very important for an individual to have a quality sex life. Your sex life is controlled by sacral chakra and can be transmuted into love and spiritual unity. If your sex energy is in a well-balanced condition, it is able to enhance and smoothen the functioning of your nervous system and the brain. Whether an individual is fertile or celibate or of adult or older age, sex chakra is extremely important.

A Portion of the sexual energy is also transmuted into high forms of pranic energy to be used in intelligent, creative, and spiritual functions. Sex energy should only be transmuted and not suppressed. Sex energy moves to upper parts of chakras including the Heart, Throat and the Crown chakras here it is transmuted into enlightenment, intelligence, kindness, love, and divine oneness.

Transformation of the sex or sacral energy into higher centers of energy and lower energies frequencies are transformed into high frequencies. Greater effectiveness and efficiency of our brains are enhanced by the transformation of pranic energy into high frequencies.

The sex or sacral chakra begins to develop at the age of 8 years, and most people's sex chakra becomes active shortly before or at puberty. During that time, your body is matured enough to procreate; you develop more awareness of the opposite sex.

The sexual organs of the female are located in the sacral chakra, and they enable her to have more emotional feelings than the male whose sexual organs are more grounded physically.

When two people who love each other engage in romantic sexual activity, their sex chakras mix and a fantastic aura are created around them.

The sex drive can be dramatically affected by the sacral chakra either negatively or positively when it's awakened. In either of these two cases, the effects are short-lived, and when the energy settles, your sex chakra is stabilized.

There several ways you can use to enhance your sexual life, one of the techniques is super brain yoga. This involves a simple and similar form of meditation for healing your sacral chakra. It requires you to sit with your back straight and to inhale deeply and to exhale gently. The major difference is that you are required to focus more on your brain as you strive to cleanse your sacral chakra.

Scientifically, an average human brain can store over one million items, and the human brain is capable of repairing the circuitry system that is broken or regenerating new neurons and brain cells caused by damage, aging or disease. Super yoga helps in keeping our brain functional and fit and it's also a good practice that can enable an aging person to counter age-related brain illnesses such as 'Alzheimer's disease and dementia. Superbrain yoga will help an individual to activate his/her brain cells. When you engage in natural sexual activity, due to focus and healing brought about by the super yoga will enable your sex energy to be easily transformed into spiritual and psychological development.

There are many other practices that you will be required to use to ensure your sexual life is enhanced and your sacral chakra is well balanced. Surrounding yourself with water is one of the most ideal options. You can even start with a simple step like having a ritual cleansing bath in your home; you can go swimming in a beach or swimming pool. Water is one of the sacral chakra's elements and can be very helpful in cleansing or unblocking the sacral chakra.

You can use meditation techniques as well. There is also the required diet to enable you to boost your sex life. Eat orange-colored foods that represent the sacral chakra and other foods like sweet potatoes, oranges, apricots, mangoes, carrots, and peaches. Also, use essential oils like Ylang Ylang and others that we had discussed earlier. Other healing techniques to boost your sex life include professional and guided Psychic healing and using healing stones.

Besides helping in the transformation of sex energy to other forms of energy, having a healthy sex life has many benefits. They will enable you to reduce tension and anxiety, making you more productive and effective. Your immune system is strengthened if your sex life is healthy and fulfilling. You will be able to defend your body against illnesses, viruses, and germs, but you should also try to eat the right diet and sleep well to maximize the benefits of a stronger immune system fully.

Healthy sex life will enable you to boost your libido and make your sex life even much pleasurable. In women, besides increasing the blood flow, it also improves vaginal lubrication and elasticity. Healthy sex life helps in stabilizing and lowering your blood pressure. For those who still don't know, sexual activity is an exercise in itself and will allow you to benefit just like a person going to a gym. Sex will help you burn calories, improve your heart rate, and increase the flow of the blood during circulation. Other benefits include improving sleep and easing stress.

Lack of pleasure in your life which is brought by sacral chakra is important for you to have a stable and good quality of life. Whether it's a sexual pleasure or enjoyment from creativeness, for instance, when you don't have a fulfilling sex life, you might experience depression, bad moods, unstable emotions, feeling lifeless or insensitiveness. Always ensure your sacral chakra is well balanced all the time.

Conclusion

Understanding ourselves as a human being is crucial in enabling us to deal with issues affecting us in our daily lives. The Chakra system does more than just helping us with our problems and goes further to enable us to have a good health and even deal with future situations or difficulties.

Using the available techniques to keep our chakras open is very important. It will help you deal with a serene and full life. You will also be able to maintain excellent relationships, develop knowledge, connect with the universe, and even connect with our spiritual being.

We have also learned the best way to learn the techniques of opening your chakras is by practicing them more regularly, creating awareness and focus while opening, healing, or balancing the chakras. When our chakra system is functioning properly, our lives are organized and all-inclusive. Also, meditating, exercising, and practicing yoga as regular as possible is generally a good idea if we wish to maintain balanced chakras and a good quality of life.

Chakras also help us with getting more integrated and feel wholeness with our lives and gain confidence that we might not have discovered we are capable of displaying when dealing with our challenges.

The book has extensively covered the topic of the chakras system and numerous ways in which it can be organized to enhance the quality of life. Besides visualization and various approaches discussed to help gain enhanced quality of life, another vital thing is the help an individual discover hidden potential which he/she can activate, utilize and gain greater fulfillment in his/her life.

Chakras Guide:

The Ultimate Beginner's Guide to Chakras and Self-Healing. Learn How to Open the Third Eye, Chakra Meditation Techniques - How to Balance Your 7 Chakras

Table of Contents

Introduction

Congratulations on purchasing *Chakras Guide: The Ultimate Beginner's Guide to Chakras and Self-Healing* and thank you for doing so. This book will teach you all you need to know about how to open your third eye, balance your 7 chakras and learn simple and effective meditation techniques to heal and cleanse your energy for good.

The following chapters will discuss all you need to know about the chakras including what and where they are, how they work and what they affect in your overall health and wellbeing on all levels. You will discover what the Seven Chakra System is and what each chakra is like in relationship to all of the others. Each chakra has its own color, frequency, qualities, characteristics and connection to your organs, glands, bodily functions, emotions, thoughts, memories and more!

Not only will you learn about the chakras and how they work with your whole body and mind, but this book will also give you perfunctory examples of how they are affected by disease, illness, and other problems we have in our health and wellness. There are plenty of ways that chakra imbalances can manifest in your life and this book wants to give you all of the tools and information you need to understand those patterns.

The practices you will learn in this book will all give you what you need to heal yourself from blockages and imbalances in your chakra system so that you can live a full, free, healthy and happy life. There are tools to help guide you including meditations and instructions on what crystals can do for you and how to use them to clear your energy and stay in balance.

If that's not enough, there's more! You will be shown 20 of the most effective mantras and affirmations that will help your energy stay in a healthy flow as you work on managing your overall chakra healing and well-being. You can see case studies of different chakra healing experiences that have given great progress to the way we learn how to look at our own chakras and heal them with these effective tools.

All of us need a way to stay in balance with our bodies, energy, mind, and feelings and this book is your ultimate guide to learning how to process the energy of chakras, open up your intuition and mental power, and find new ways to create abundance in your life.

There are plenty of books on this subject on the market, thanks again for choosing this one! Every effort was made to ensure it is full of as much useful information as possible, please enjoy!

Chapter 1: Explaining the Chakras

All over the world and all over the internet, people are talking about chakras: what they are, what they do, and why we should all know about them and how they work. The chakras are not new to our modern culture and have had a long history in other cultures, providing a lot of knowledge to the way Eastern cultures have practiced healing and medicine for the past 3,000 to 4,000 years.

If you are new to learning about chakras, that's great! You came to the right place because this book is a basic guide to give you all of the information you need to understand the chakras and what they are to each and every one of us.

In this chapter, you will learn what they are, how we discovered their existence, and who has them and can heal them. Together, we will go through the journey of awakening the chakras and I will be your guide on your journey to self-healing through your chakra system. To get you started, let's ask a simple question:

What Are Chakras?

Chakras are energy. In each of our body systems, there is an energetic layer that you may have heard a little bit about already. Have you ever heard of auras? People describe being able to see or read the colorful light, or energy that emanates outside of people. There are even certain types of photography that can capture the auric field so you can see what it looks like.

Chakras are the same type of energy and the two systems are actually a part of the same whole. Chakras are a field of energy that vibrates at certain frequencies in your body. When you are going about your everyday life, you won't even notice that energy, because we aren't shown or taught how to understand them or work with healing them when we are young.

Every day, your chakras are a part of your life experience. The energy that they are is something that cannot be seen with the naked eye by most people (although some healers are known to have pictured them) and they are always in some kind of fluctuation between high and low, or negative and positive energy.

The chakras have been described as being vortexes, or "wheels" of spinning energy that have a color and a light frequency associated with them. They are working hard to keep your health in order and when you are not in good health, neither are your chakras. Let me explain a little bit more about how energy works so that you can understand how the chakras work with our whole experience of life.

Energy is in all things. Everything has an energetic force field or vibrational frequency that can actually be measured with technology. We are energy, the device you are holding in your hand is energy. The chair you are sitting on has an energetic output. Everything has energy. When you are thinking about the chakras, and you can picture them as energy, try seeing how that energy can shift or change in certain ways.

If you are feeling really great on a sunny day, feeling the energy of the sun and the flowers in bloom and then all of a sudden it gets cloudy and the energy changes and there is electricity in the air because of a storm, the energy of everything changes as a result. The same is true of your chakra energy. When you are in a healthy balance and in good health and then you suffer a horrible blow or difficult life experience that causes pain, grief and loss, your energy changes, and so does your chakra system.

Another way to think about energy is with magnets. Have you ever played with two magnets and felt the push or the pull in both of them when you try to put them together? On one side the magnets have an eagerness to come together and will force closeness, slamming together, while on the opposite side, they will push each other apart and are impossible to touch together. It's quite exciting to see and feel.

Chakras can behave in the same way with other people, experiences, health problems, and so forth. They can also become blocked, deficient or excessive in their "energetic flow" or vibration. It's like a clogged sink, or drain; the water can't flow down because there is something in the way and until you remove the obstruction, the sink stays clogged.

The energy of the chakras works in a similar way: if you have an illness, emotional wounds, trauma, chronic pain, and so on, you may have a blocked chakra, or more than one, that cannot function properly, like a clogged drain.

So basically, the chakras are your energy centers in your body that are always where a lot of your emotional, mental, physical and spiritual issues are stored. Anything that isn't properly healed, balanced and resolved will stay stuck in the chakra and create long term, or chronic issues that will cause you unnecessary difficulty in life.

As you learn more about how we discovered them and what they represent, you will know more about what it can do for you to help them heal, balance and flow freely to rejuvenate your life.

How Did We Discover Them?

Chakras are not new. We have always had this energy circling inside of us. We just didn't know it was there until sometime during the time of the Buddha, and possibly before, dating back to 1200 to 400 BCE. The Buddha existed sometime between 563 and 400 BCE. When he was on his spiritual quest, he described the element of enlightenment and awakening as part of a system of energy that rotates within us at all times, that when opened and aligned will lead to spiritual awakening of the self and the soul.

You don't have to be Buddhist to believe in these concepts, and it actually wasn't only the Buddha who described these concepts. Others across the world, at the same and different times, talked of similar energies in the body. Even in the Bible, the miracles of healing that were written about were spoken of as if they had all to do with an unseen life force or energy that came from God.

The truth is, that energy is in all of us, and that is what was written in the ancient Hindu religious texts known as the Vedas. This compendium of spiritual doctrine and documentation described these energy vortices and named then chakras, which translates to mean "wheel or circle". In other interpretations of Indo-European languages, it translates to mean "turn".

Several different cultures over time have had a different description of this energy system. In Traditional Chinese Medicine, this energy is known as Chi and is a part of acupuncture and Tai Chi. Although it appears differently in that system it describes the same kind of connection between this energetic, inner-force, and all of the systems of the body.

The chakra system that we are talking about in this book is the one described by the ancient Hindu religions that explored and explained the concept in great detail, involving it in all of their practices of healing and internal balance, including the invention of yoga and the practices of eating certain foods and herbs to heal the specific energy imbalances that can occur for a variety of reasons across a lifetime.

There are a lot of different methods for healing the chakras that have come out of this origin and discovery, yoga and ayurvedic diets being one of them. Others include crystal healing, Reiki, vibrational healing methods (sound baths), meditation, acupuncture, Tai Chi, and many more!

The question is: can you heal your chakras on your own?

Are We All Able to Heal Our Own?

Yes! The answer is an unequivocal yes. Many people have a belief that you cannot take your health and healing into your own hands and that you need an expert or five to tell you how to heal your own issues. In many cases, we do need healthcare professionals to help us with a wide range of physical, mental and emotional issues. And on that note, here is an important disclaimer to read before you go any further:

DISCLAIMER: If you are in need of medical attention or experiencing any kind of medical emergency, please see a medical, or health care professional.

Healing the chakras is definitely something you can accomplish on your own with the tools I am going to show you in this book, but you may also need to treat some conditions with the help of a doctor or professional healer. There are other ways that you can help heal your chakras that incorporate a variety of techniques and as you continue your journey through these pages, you will have a clearer idea of what I mean.

The healing journey you take is unique to you and your energy. Everyone's chakra healing experience will be different and if you feel excited to take a look at the different ways you can begin this wild path of discovery, then please keep reading!

You have the power to heal your chakras and there are ways that you can begin this journey on your own as you find other modalities to work with along the journey. A few of the ways you will learn about healing your chakras in this book include:

- Meditations
- Crystal Therapy
- Mantras
- Creative Visualization
- Diet and Movement
- Awareness

Anything that you do to directly focus on your inner life-force and how it is affecting your life will bring you into a deeper connection to your wholeness and abundance. The rest of this book is going to teach you everything you need to know about how the chakras work, the benefits of healing them, issues that can come up, and methods for taking control of your own healing journey through your chakra system.

Chapter 2: The Seven Chakra System

The Seven Chakra system is where the journey begins. The whole story behind the processes of the body can be learned through understanding each chakra and what they are representative of in your system. All of your chakras will ascend from the base of the spine up to the crown of the head. Each chakra has an elemental power and strength, as well as several qualities and properties that are specific to the region of the body they are located in.

The following sections will give you the details of each chakra, starting at the base of the spine and going all the way up to the top of the head. Before we look at the chakras individually, let's explore the system as a whole.

The chakras are aligned together in one unified force of energy. Each one connects to the next and with all of them responsive to each other through this link and connection, if one works against itself, that means that others will compensate. The whole system exists as an internal essence that some people call 'spirit'. The spirit energy of you is what aligns you with your highest vibrational frequency and purpose. This is what causes us to search for healing and ask the higher questions about why we are all here and what we are made of.

The beginning of your life was pure. When you first come into the world, your energy is basic and simple; it has not yet been complicated by emotional problems, illness, patterning and thought programs given to you by your parents and caregivers, as well as society and culture.

As we grow older, we absorb information in the form of energy. Everything we take in as information is energy that contributes to our overall reality and experience of life. When you look at a kindergartner, they are learning how to perceive language through lines and numbers, letters and words. They are also just starting to understand social behaviors and the influences of poor behavior versus good behavior.

All of this "energetic information" goes through your whole system, not just your brain. It happens to your chakras as well, and the information you are taught will incorporate itself into the energy of the seven chakras, telling you how to exist in this world.

When we are older, we are sometimes overly affected by our past programming, which results in a need to transform and improve the self. Energy is the answer to working on that practice and here is why: every struggle you have in your life that comes from within you is based on the Seven Chakra System and how well it is functioning.

The chakras are our equalizer and balancing system and they are each affected by the food you eat, the people you are involved with, your beliefs about the world and yourself, and a variety of other platforms.

Let's take a look at the Seven Chakras individually and give you a bigger perspective on what they all say about your energy.

1. The Root Chakra

The Root chakra is the first chakra. It sits at the base of the spine in the area of the tail bone. The root chakra is associated with certain fears, emotions, dilemmas, and issues as it is always working hard to keep you grounded and secure, like the roots of a tree. It is the color red and is associated with the element of earth.

The energy of this area is connected to your legs down to your feet. People with thigh, knee, or foot issues can have systemic problems in the root chakra. Your legs and feet are what support your body. It is the structure that holds you upright and makes you feel secure and if your root energy is out of balance, you can feel off-balance as well. It is also connected to the Adrenal Cortex and issues of that system.

Security, survival, and groundedness are the issues of the root. All of your energy in this area circles around your wealth in finances, your ability to make ends meet, your structure and stability, and your choices for keeping yourself healthy and alive. This chakra can also be associated with issues of karmic retribution and past life trauma, as well as repressed childhood issues and emotions.

2. The Sacral Chakra

The sacral chakra is in the next position up the spine and rests within the pelvic girdle where the sacrum brings together the two iliac bones. It is the color orange and is associated with the element of water. This chakra is connected to the vibration of sexual energy and reproduction.

The matters of fertility, virility and sexual drive are found most frequently in this chakra. It is therefore connected to the sexual organs (ovaries and testicles), as well as the bladder, and lower intestines. Imbalances in your sacral chakra can have a direct impact on the functionality of these organ systems.

Creativity, passion, desire, emotional balance, and sexuality are all a part of a thriving sacral chakra.

3. The Solar Plexus Chakra

The solar plexus chakra is above the sacral chakra, positioned above the belly button. It is the color yellow and is connected to the element of fire. This chakra pertains to your digestion and adrenal glands. Any imbalances and issues in these systems will be caused by, or connected to blocked and unhealthy chakra energy here.

This area pertains to personal power, vitality, drive, and ambition. It relates to how you use or process energy in your life, and also how you present yourself to the world. Self-esteem is closely linked to this area, as well as aggressiveness and being overbearing.

Anything having to do with the fiery energy of yourself and how you are in all that you do, alone or in a group, revolves around this area. It can be a sign of excessive energy when a person is aggressive, and a sign of deficiency in energy when someone is sheepish or shy.

4. The Heart Chakra

The heart chakra is in the chest area around the physical heart and is related to all matter of the heart as well. This chakra is green and connected to the element of air. Anyone with a heart problem or issues with their blood or lymphatic circulation is likely to have an imbalance in this chakra. The thymus gland, which regulates immunity and also produces hormones.

Emotions of love are strongly represented here and anything relating to partnership, friendship, group and community love and bonding, and spiritual love will be related to this energy center. People who are overly emotional, or incredibly closed off and emotionally cold, will have some imbalances in this chakra.

The heart chakra is an opening and gateway to bridge the energies of the lower and upper chakras. The lower chakras are about more earthly realities while the upper chakras pertain more to spiritual growth, ethereal matters and enlightenment. The heart is the mid-point between these two realities and is an open door to connect you to both sides of life.

5. The Throat Chakra

The throat chakra is at the base of the neck and is connected to the voice and the breath, as well as the ability to make a sound. It is the color blue and is associated with the element of sound and vibration. It connects to hearing and listening as much as it connects to speaking and vocalizing.

This chakra connects to the vocal cords, lungs, neck and thyroid gland. The thyroid produces hormones that are responsible for regulating metabolism, digestive functions, brain development, heart function and overall maintenance of various systems.

The throat is where your personal truth is spoken and where we are able to verbally communicate. It is connected to self-expression, listening, and the ability to communicate well and truthfully.

6. The Brow (Third Eye) Chakra

The brow chakra is more commonly known as the third eye and sits centered in the forehead just above the eyebrows. It is the color indigo and is connected to the element of light. This is where people are able to 'see' in their mind's eye and what is called the 'seat of psychic awareness and vision'.

This chakra relates to the central nervous system, left eye, pituitary gland, nasal cavity, and cerebellum. The thyroid functions to secrete hormones into your bloodstream. All of these systems are linked to mental function, and hormone balance as well as clairvoyance and psychic abilities.

There are many people who very hard to open this chakra as fast as they can because of the desire to practice a 'higher' psychic sense. As it happens, this is one of the more difficult chakras to balance and open and requires the effort of healing many of the other chakras first, before you can fully awaken the third eye (see Chapter 4 for more information on opening the third eye chakra).

7. The Crown Chakra

The seventh chakra is at the top of the head, right at the area of the crown and is named for this position. It is the color violet and is connected to the element of ether. You can easily confuse this chakra with the 6th (brow) chakra because they are so physically close, and because they assume a similar point of opening, awakening, and enlightenment.

It is connected to the right eye, cerebrum, and pineal gland which regulates circadian rhythm and sleep cycles. It is also assumed to be the center of spiritual wisdom and has been celebrated as such by many cultures for many centuries.

The crown chakra relates to awakening the mind to know more about the Universe and the collective unity consciousness. It pertains to the regular opening and processing of energies in all its forms in everyday life to receive more connection to your own purpose and spiritual wisdom.

These 7 chakras function as individual parts of a whole and can be seen separately, but it must be understood that work together to form the ultimate balance. You can't heal one without waking up and inspiring another one to shift and transform. They are like Rube Goldberg Machines: when you set one thing into motion, it causes a series of endless cause and effect events.

In addition to these 7 chakras, there are also energy wheels in the palms of each hand, the soles of each foot, and outside the top of the head above the crown chakra. They are not something that will directly affect the endocrine and organ systems or your physical or emotional state, but they are important to be aware of for self-healing practices.

In the next chapter, you will discover more about awakening the 7 chakras and what it means to go on that journey of healing and balancing.

Chapter 3: Awakening the 7 Chakras

When you are available to ask yourself what you want out of your healing journey, you can welcome the reality of what it means to truly heal. There are a lot of possibilities for how your chakra imbalances will show up in your life and may have been so ingrained in your reality for such a long time, that you don't even realize that there are even any issues, to begin with.

What you get out of this experience of healing is entirely up to you and your personal goals with wellness and life happiness. Presence with your energy system and awareness of your specific healing goals is what will help you begin to question what needs healing the most in your life. For some it may be a physical issue; for others, it might be an emotional problem. Whatever your purpose for wanting to find a new method for healing, the results of your progress will be noticeable over a period of time.

So, what does it mean to awaken the chakras anyway? The chakras, as you have read, are all energy wheels in your body and they are always working in accordance with your overall life experience. When you are used to living a certain way, eating certain foods, working a certain line of work, going about your life with certain patterns, behaviors, and beliefs, your chakras are energetically cooperative to what you are showing them every day.

This means that if you are a chain smoker or an addict to some kind of substance, your energy will focus on only knowing that reality because it is what you are always wanting to give to it energetically. If you were to stop smoking or quit an addiction, your energy would almost immediately begin to shift to incorporate another kind of energy and it will probably be a more positive vibrational frequency.

Awakening the chakras involves a long-term healing program that you have to open yourself to as you seek to know another level of healing, transformation, and growth. When you start with some of these basic chakra healing techniques, you will begin to unravel some of the realities of how it can feel to open these doors and purge some of the issues that are stored in these parts of your system.

It can be a difficult experience if you are not sure what is happening, but if you are aware of the goal of healing and some of the things that can happen through chakra awakening, then you may be able to find it less uncomfortable. You are also likely to experience intense feelings of joy, harmony, and bliss during an energy transformation, so it isn't all difficult, all of the time.

Essentially, chakra awakening is when you begin to start the sequence of shifting your energy centers so that they can readjust over time and begin to recalibrate your frequency so that you are living in a higher vibration. When you start your process, there are a lot of things that can occur and here are a few things that can begin to happen as a result of opening your energy for healing and balance:

- Painful memories and traumatic experiences, even as far back as early childhood and infancy can begin to surface

- Visions and altered dream states have been reported by many people

- Fluctuations in energy, either being overly fatigued and tired or having inexhaustive energy to do a lot more

- Change in attitudes or beliefs as your mental programming begins to shift

- Appetite fluctuations, as well as cravings for certain foods or beverages

- Emotional release in the form of crying, laughing, anger or frustration, often out of the blue

- Difficulty sleeping, or restlessness

- Humming, tingling, or buzzing sensation in the body

- Temperature fluctuations from hot to cold, back and forth

- The onset of cold or flu-like symptoms revolving around energetic purging and cleansing in the chakras

- Achiness in the muscles, bones, and joints

- Feelings of gratitude and compassion that feel overwhelming

- Expressions of great joy and feelings of abundance and prosperity

- Feelings of depression or heartache as a result of repressed emotions coming up to the surface for healing

- Life changes as in changing careers, moving to new cities, going overseas, taking a journey

- Significant relationships starting or ending

- Emotional highs and lows

- Physical practices changing, going from a sedentary lifestyle, to suddenly having an urge to exercise or practice other healing practices, like yoga, walking, or swimming

- Participation in new hobbies and community activities

- Finding a new life purpose or passion to explore

- And more!

The list seems endless because there are so many ways that awakening the chakras can influence your life. As it happens, your body, mind, and spirit will work to repossess the original frequency that you had when you were a newborn baby. This was what you came into the world knowing as your original frequency and as you begin to grow, you receive the energy of the whole world, everyone around you, and all of the things that you are taught to know and believe.

This includes being shown how to eat food, or what is worth your time and energy, as well as how to worship and believe in something, or what you should be when you grow up. As a result of early life conditioning and programming, some of us may lose sight of original cause to be here and we go through our lives with a whole lot of other energy that we don't need, blocking our chakras.

Practices in working with chakra alignment have come into existence over the centuries and have continued to be utilized today to help many people reach their personal and private goals of awakening to the self and healing the energies from within. As you look forward to beginning this journey it is important to know some of the following things:

- Chakra awakening takes time and is different for everyone.

- Not all problems and issues can be resolved with these techniques alone; some issues may require the aid of a doctor, therapist, health coach, yoga teacher, Reiki master, acupuncturist and others.

- All of the energy of your chakra system is unique to you and your personal tone of frequency and vibration. We are not all supposed to look alike, sound alike, and have the exact same chakra healing results.

- Generations of human beings have been looking for answers for how to heal the whole self and chakras are a part of the healing path.

- All of us have a chakra system and most of us are in a great imbalance most of the time.

- Awakening the chakras requires a consistent devotion and dedication if you are truly interested in making healing progress.

- You can always resolve your energy issues with focus and concentration, but they are never going to ask you to heal them; you have to choose to do the work.

- The chakras are a practice associated with other healing pearls of wisdom, such as yoga, Ayurveda, Reiki and more. Utilizing these practices in addition to what you will learn in this book will result in a faster progression of healing.

- Awakening the chakras is powerful and you will feel it on all levels: physical, mental, emotional, and spiritual.

- Awareness of all life and all matter will help you see more of your own possibilities as you are going through your healing experience.

- Ways to help you accept a deeper connection to your healing path will involve working with your intuition and benefiting from your own knowledge about how to move forward through your experience.

- You can work in whatever ways feel the best to you and are in control of your healing journey.

- Awakening is significant and will change your life, so it helps to know that you are ready to pursue that course of action.

- Chakra awakening leads to a life of personal power, open-heartedness, creativity, passion, dedication, speaking the truth, trusting your wisdom, and feeling connected to the whole of the Universe.

All of these points are here to show you some of the ways you can expect to move ahead easily. As you have read, the chakras are not only energy centers; they connect to your vital organs, your endocrine system, your emotional states and moods, your belief systems and values, and your level of overall health.

As you go forward through these chapters, ask yourself where you are feeling out of balance in your life and consider what you might start to awaken as you move forward on your healing path. When you are able to open your third eye, you will just know what to do and where to practice rebalancing and healing in your body centers. The main point of learning to heal yourself is to get to a place where you can hear and feel what your body is trying to show you. An open third eye will help you continue your chakra healing journey by showing you how to stay in balance and how to live a life of personal truth.

In the next chapter, you will discover more about how to awaken and open the third eye to experience higher levels of healing and attaining your life goals.

Chapter 4: How to Open Your Third Eye

Your third eye is your inner vision and psychic wisdom. Not all people are able to look through it and see clearly and you are not going to get very far in your personal awakening if you don't believe that it is possible to have these kinds of experiences. What are the things you are likely to experience with an open third eye?

- An ability to enhance your psychic perception

- Sensing or knowing things are going to happen before they do

- Profound and prophetic dreams or visions

- Clear insight and wisdom, as if a light bulb has gone on in your mind

- A significant increase in the ability to understand bigger life matters and concepts, such as 'why are we all here', etc.

- Feelings of intensity in certain situations because you are able to 'see' more than what is shown (ex: perceiving other people's emotions well, or knowing what happened right before you walked into the room without explanation)

- Having a clearer view of your own well-being and state of health

- Clairvoyance and claircognizance

- Channeling guidance and wisdom from other sources (i.e., spirit guides)

These are just some of the common ways that an open third chakra can start to manifest in your life. Of course, we are all capable of knowing reality in this way, and not everyone will because of imbalances in the chakras, blocks in energy, or a refusal to accept these possibilities as a realistic lifestyle.

Opening the third is not the first step of chakra awakening, but it can be a goal for many people who are eager to get to this level of personal enlightenment. It can take years of practice to get to this level of awakening with your third eye and many people will struggle against it because of how different it feels to become that 'aware' when a majority of your life has existed in another way.

You are always able to speed up the process when you are consistently working with your chakra system to create a healthy level of balance and vibration. You can think of it like going to your daily yoga class, or as a part of your weekly meditations and personal care regimen. Tending to the energy system of your body is a part of how everything else is functioning and the more you work toward keeping it in a good state of health, the easier it will become to open and awaken new levels of awareness.

In order to open the third eye, you will most likely have to work toward a system or approach that can help your whole system, such as the one you are learning about in this book. Healing the chakras works on all levels and so it isn't something that happens overnight or in a few weeks or months; it is an ongoing journey that you will experience and explore for the rest of your life.

There are a few things to consider as you prepare to open your third eye and they are:

- Predicting your future isn't something you are able to do easily; it has to come with a significant amount of practice and wisdom.

- Issues of pride and ego are something that must be healed in this chakra before it will open all the way.

- Blockages and imbalances will remain here if you have intentions of maliciousness or manipulation with this type of gift.

- The lower chakras are just as important to understanding how to have balance in your third eye and so healing these areas, in correlation to your psychic work, will make it happen faster and more easily.

- Your third eye needs to be grounded by your earthly self' it can be easy to let go of your life reality to live in your vision state, but it will send other areas of your life into turmoil if you are not paying attention to everything else.

- Teaching yourself when to use your third eye is a part of the journey; it won't always work with everything you are experiencing because you will need to have experiences on other levels (i.e., heart level, sacral level, etc.).

Asking yourself some questions about your intentions for knowing this level of energetic opening will lead you to want to know how to connect to that understanding even more. Once you feel opening begin to occur here, you will actually know what people have been looking for through enlightenment for centuries. It is no easy task and it will take you on quite the journey as it is happening over time.

What are some of the ways you can open your third eye? The following list will give you some answers about what you can do to open this chakra:

1. Spend time in reflection and contemplation.

2. Practice silence so that you can better listen to your third eye.

3. Meditate daily and include a focus on and visualization of your third eye opening while you chant your chosen mantra.

4. Keep a dream journal and start a practice of lucid dreaming.

5. Eat lighter foods, or go on a juice cleanse.

6. Ground yourself while you explore the upper chakras.

7. Use a crystal on your third eye. You can lie down on the floor and place the crystal on top of your forehead to help you really clear and balance this energy. (See Chapter 13 for more details)

8. Practice your intuitive abilities with conscious effort.

9. Using Breathing techniques to enliven the brain.

10. Connect to your creativity and imagination; 'daydream'.

Any and all of these tools will work and they work best when practiced together regularly. Very few things in this world can be arrived at in one attempt at it and as with opening your third eye, it will require some consistent focus and practice.

In addition to these ten steps, working with your other chakras, to help them come into better alignment and balance, will be a necessary aspect of working with your open third eye. Remember, the system is a whole and each chakra asks for balance so that they can all work well as one life-force.

It isn't hard to open your third eye. All it takes is the choice to make it happen and these steps and pointers to help you handle the experience well. You don't need anything to open your third eye; you just need your own body, mind, and spirit and the choice to know and to see beyond the limits of your mind.

Chapter 5: Troubleshooting Chakra Awakening: Things to Avoid

We can all get a little carried away in a practice or a process. We can get lazy and not put in as much effort as we should. There are always fluctuations with life because we need to be flexible when the unexpected occurs. When you are going through a chakra awakening experience it will be very 'eye-opening' and transformative. As a lot of people are discovering these tools and methods and choosing to align with higher consciousness, there are several reports available of what many people have encountered in their own experiences.

For a lot of us, it is an amazing and powerful shift and rediscovery that can turn your life upside down and help you to work on the life path and goals you are actually wishing for, rather than living the life you thought you had to for whatever reasons. Using your intuition to guide you along the way can help, but it won't always be accessible and here's why: when you are in an awakening experience, you are dealing with your past and your present problems so that you can invest in a greater future.

Your processing experience is what will have to happen in order for you to be able to live in value to your chakra energies. What this means is that you will have to enjoy the turmoil of poking your internal hornet's nest, so to speak. Whatever you are going through right now, today has likely had a connection to the energy of your past that has been locked into your 7 chakras. In order to find your way into a new balance, you will have to see, know, feel and sense things that might have caused you pain in the past that are presently manifesting as other issues, like chronic pain, chronic fatigue syndrome, hormone imbalances, depression or anxiety, and so on.

There are ways that you can help yourself have a smoother, lighter, and more carefree and joyful journey as you stimulate the negative energies that you are working to let go of and purge. Troubleshooting chakra awakening is a part of the process that will help you to stay grounded and putting your best intentions and focus on healing.

The following list provides you with some key points about what you should avoid or be aware of as you go through the purging and cleansing experience.

1. Avoid processed foods, as well as high sugar content foods and drinks, alcohol, and drugs. All of these chemicals have a powerful interaction with your energy and your vital organ systems. If you actually want to heal your chakras and your whole body, then you may have to make some significant changes in your diet and nutrition.

2. Avoid attitudes and behaviors that will perpetuate bad habits and negativity. Seek to have a more positive outlook and be open to letting go of patterns that cause you to feel unhealthy.

3. Avoid situations, people and environments that feel 'toxic' to you. There are a lot of scenarios that are unhealthy for people and sometimes we just go along with it because we feel like we have to. Part of stimulating a healing process and purging the negativity in our bodies is the letting go of particular

people, places or activities that keep us feeling 'off' in our world.

4. Avoid participating in anything that causes you physical or emotional harm or pain. Some events in life are unavoidable and we cannot control everything, but we can control some things and if you are repeatedly offering yourself something painful, it will cost your healing journey and cause it to take a lot longer.

5. Avoid extremes. Extremes could be anything like binge-watching television for several days in a row, to drinking to excess, to uprooting and changing your job or living situation out of nowhere. These things may be tempting and are often coping mechanisms when we are uncomfortable with our awakening experiences. Looking for healthier ways to process is a much better action for the chakras.

6. Process your opening with a healthy diet, sleep practice, hydration, and quality of life that will feel supportive and compatible with how you are going through your chakra awakening.

7. Explore alternative methods for health care, like yoga, acupuncture, Reiki, massage, lymphatic drainage, sound baths, and deprivation tanks. All of these methods are ways that you can connect more deeply to the process of helping your chakra energy shift and heal. Self-care is a huge problem in our culture; most people have not learned how to make it a regular part of everyday life.

8. Arrange for space to be alone and have quiet, reflective moments. It doesn't have to be a meditation or a specific practice; it can simply be having solitude and journaling or contemplating what your present feelings or state of mind is.

9. Develop daily routines and habits that support your chakra awakening and healing journey. You don't have to do everything all at once; that would be too extreme. Start slowly and change one thing at a time to include more healthy energy healing practices.

10. Be patient and kind to yourself. This awakening experience is about you and your life and how you want to live well. It can be easy to go overboard and feel unhappy with your progress, or like you aren't doing enough. That kind of belief or attitude will just cause even more negative energy for you to release, purge and heal, and so it is best to help yourself feel well along the journey.

All of these types of things can take time to find balance with and incorporate into a new lifestyle and routine. It's never easy to just change everything all at once and that is why it is best to plan for a long road to travel and that as you slowly start making some changes your chakras will start to change with you.

One of the biggest issues that we all have in our modern age is instant gratification. Everyone wants a miracle cure, or easy fix to a lot of problems or life issues and the number one way that people fall off the chakra awakening wagon is to give up and stay with their lower vibrational energy because it is easy, familiar, and it doesn't require any hard work.

Awakening your chakras isn't hard, especially if you are wanting to create a more balanced and healthy life. It can actually be a joyful and pleasurable experience for a person to experience and as long as you have that attitude about it going in, you are likely to have a much better time hanging in there when things feel a little rough around the edges.

One major aspect of this practice is that you will have to go over it on a daily or regular basis in order to make the really big, positive changes and shifts. If you are not ready to make that a part of your life habits, then you may need more time to do some research and mentally prepare for the possibilities of making so much change in your life.

So, here are some additional tips to help you stay focused and avoid issues that may come up along the road:

- Make time for you.

- Make time for healing work, such as meditation, yoga, Reiki, etc.

- Help yourself by changing what isn't good for you (food, alcohol, lack of exercise).

- Practice daily, or regularly.

- Have patience and compassion for yourself.

- Pay attention to your intuition and let it help you make wise decisions about your healing path.

- Let go of the things in your life that are causing you pain, harm, or misfortune.

- Demand space for your growth and awakening.

- Get plenty of good rest and sleep.

- Keep yourself hydrated.

- Accept that change is inevitable and that nothing is permanent.

You can really help yourself open a lot more quickly and pleasantly when you are practicing healthy choices and working with your intuition as you go. There are certainly times where we will not have space for these exercises or energy clearing methods and that's okay. Life is full of ups and downs, ebbs and flows. There will be plenty of opportunities throughout your chakra awakening experience when you will need to just go with the flow.

- Avoid being rigid and overbearing with your healing experience.

- Avoid engineering impossible goals pertaining to your energy awakening.

- Avoid criticizing your lack of movement forward, especially if you need to just hold space for an important part of your healing work and give time to resettle and transform your energy.

- Avoid living in doubt or fear that you won't be able to do this work and just let it come forward in the right moments for you.

- Avoid boxing yourself into only one way of going through chakra awakening. The experience will be unique to you, so trust your intuition.

Anything that comes up along the way is likely meant to help you resolve some of the physical, mental, and emotional issues that have been a part of your blocked chakra system. It is absolutely normal for there to be strong feelings and emotions surfacing along the way. It is also partly true that things might get a little worse before they start to feel better.

When you are releasing serious illness, trauma, and old wounds from years ago, it can take some time to process and release; but, don't worry! As long as you are taking good care of yourself, trusting your intuition, avoiding things that will set you back, and making space for healing, you will be in good standing and the process will go that much more quickly for you.

Engage with the positive ways you can manage and maintain your chakra awakening experience and prepare to be amazed at how exciting it is to transform through healing your chakras.

The next chapter will go into more specific detail about what the physical, emotional, mental, and spiritual imbalances can be within your chakra system. You will read through each chakra again, from the root to the crown, to understand each one's imbalances within these categories of self-expression.

Chapter 6: Physical, Emotional and Mental Imbalances and How to Heal Them

The seven main chakras, as you have read, are all connected to a certain level in the body, as well as a specific organ system, gland secretion, emotional quality, mental perspective, and spiritual thought. Not all of us have deeper struggles with these parts of ourselves and many people don't even need to go through this kind of work in order to feel what they want to in their lives. That isn't to say that they don't have energy imbalances in their chakras; everyone will have that throughout the course of their life. It's more about knowing that it is different for everyone and everyone's body.

You have already learned some of the knowledge you need to understand the chakras and what they represent in relation to your whole system of life. This chapter will specifically talk about the various imbalances that can occur in each of the following categories: physical, mental, emotional, and spiritual.

There are a lot of ways that an individual person will experience these imbalances, so keep that in mind as you are taking in this information. You may notice something in these sections that will ring true for you, but perhaps you are feeling it in a different category, or in a different chakra, and that's okay.

The point is that you get a general overview of what can be the result of imbalanced chakras so that you know where you are needing to go for purging, cleansing, and rebalancing your energy.

1. <u>**The Root Chakra**</u>

Physical

The Adrenal Cortex is the part of the endocrine system connected to the root chakra. It is all about the fight or flight survival mentality. It makes sense, then, that this root area would be concerned with qualities of survival and security.

Eating disorders are commonplace with this chakra imbalance, such as anorexia or bulimia. Obesity is also connected to this chakra. Some other issues are forms of arthritis, auto-immune diseases, problems with the spine, hips, knees, legs, and feet, chronic fatigue syndrome, and various forms of cancer.

This chakra is about physical energy and power. It is connected to the part of you that can sprint away from a hungry tiger, or lift a car off of someone with super-human strength. It is a survival instinct.

Mental

Mental imbalances in the root chakra can look like a need to always think about money or finances. If you are insecure in your life due to blocked root chakra energy, you may always think about making more money, or needing to have more of something in your life, not necessarily money. This is also a place where you may have thoughts of self-worth or a lack of self-worth. You may have a lot of trust issues and are less likely to trust new people, wary of anyone who might 'uproot' you, especially when you are already feeling unstable.

Emotional

Emotional imbalances here look like nervousness, fear, and anxiety. A lot of the thoughts and emotions are connected and so you may be feeling either greedy and materialistic if you have excessive root chakra energy, or you will feel unwelcome, insecure, and unstable if it is under-active. You may have feelings of being resistant to change and your obsession, or fear, is security.

Spiritual

This is the chakra of karmic retribution. All that means is that you are carrying the wounds or deeds of past lives inside of this energy to be healed in this lifetime. Your cycles of life will represent opportunities for you to make those healing strides, or not, depending on your interest to change.

This is also where we store a majority of our deeper childhood wounds, fears, and traumas.

2. <u>The Sacral Chakra</u>

Physical

The ovaries and testicles are the glands in the endocrine system that are connected to the sacral chakra. They are responsible for the secretion of the hormones testosterone and estrogen and are related to procreation, as well as the energy of being male or female.

Other organs connected to this system are the bladder, uterus, and prostate. Physical issues that are the result of sacral chakra imbalances can involve bladder problems, like incontinence and urinary tract infections. Reproductive issues like infertility in women and sterility in men are not uncommon, as well as a lack of sex drive, or frigidity. It can also represent an overactive sex drive which is an excess of energy in this chakra.

Other issues are kidney and gall stones, prostate and vaginal cancers, diseases of the pelvis, and anything relating to the lower intestine and bowels.

Mental

Creativity is a huge part of this chakra and so if you are lacking imagination or an ability to create anything, even just an interesting meal, you may have some imbalances in this chakra. Thoughts of desire or lack of desire are related to this area. It is the chakra of sexuality and feeling and so it has a tendency to be more of emotional space. This can be represented in your thoughts as thinking you are too emotional, or that you are not trying hard enough to meet other people for relationship purposes.

Emotional

An overactive sacral chakra might mean that you are expressing yourself in an over-emotional way all of the time. You might also get easily attached to people and can be very sexual, or very easily disrupted on an emotional level.

On the other hand, if you are deficient, or underactive in the sacral chakra energy, then you are more likely to have a more stoic, stiff and unemotional approach to life, letting very few feelings speak for you at any given moment. The balance lies in having an openness without being overly emotional.

Spiritual

This is the energy of the artist. It is where your creativity lies and so from a spiritual perspective, it is your deepest connection to creative energy and the natural flow of artistic expression, passion, and desire. Those with an imbalance here may feel like their life is bland, indifferent and not very colorful or exciting.

3. The Solar Plexus Chakra

Physical

The Pancreas is the endocrine gland responsible for secretions of insulin which helps to regulate metabolism. If you are suffering from any insulin production issues, or related issues, like Diabetes, this will be related to the solar plexus chakra. Hypoglycemia, illness of the adrenal organs, and digestive problems are of concern.

The digestive system is about how you integrate nutrients and store it or utilize it as energy, thusly the solar plexus chakra ends up being directly linked to power, as well as control. To have a healthy diet, we must exercise some self-control. The upper intestines, back, and spine are also connected to this chakra, so having any kind of chronic issue with these body areas will be under the domain of the third chakra.

Mental

This chakra has a lot to do with the Ego-mind and the way that we see ourselves, or how we relate to groups. There are a lot of issues of self-esteem and self-worth and the balance of being confident without being excessively confident, or egomaniacal.

There can also be a lot of aggressive attitudes or behaviors with regard to an overactive solar plexus, and conversely, attitudes of passiveness and timidity in the underactive chakra. Either way, the thoughts are out of balance with the self and the other chakras.

Emotional

If you feel like you are not enough, or if you have an issue of significant low self-esteem, you may express that emotion all of the time without even realizing it. Emotions like social-anxiety, fear of being judged or criticized, placating others so you can be considered valuable to them, circling around sensitivity to your own needs without ever fulfilling them, and so on, can be represented in an imbalanced solar plexus. Those who are domineering have feelings that they are better than everyone around them, and under the surface, they are actually compensating for even lower self-esteem and lack of self-worth. The pendulum will usually always swing both ways with every chakra.

Spiritual

This is the spiritual reality of 'I am'. This represents your right to be here and to exist in your fullness and wholeness as an individual confidently. Spiritually, this can involve a lot of work for someone who thinks or feels that they are not allowed to be themselves, or that they have to be themselves so much that they end up steamrolling other people.

The identity is a large part of the spiritual journey and how you fit into the greater whole of all things. This chakra, when out of balance, will ask you to compensate for your true self by acting like someone you are not as a way to fit into the group.

4. <u>The Heart Chakra</u>

Physical

The heart chakra is connected to the thymus gland in the endocrine system which produces lymphocytes. These cells are directly linked to our immune function and ability to have strong health and wellness overall. The heart chakra is also related to issues of the heart, cardiovascular tissues and blood.

Some of the resulting issues are high or low blood pressure, circulation issues, arrhythmia, cancer, and some involuntary muscle issues. The lungs are also connected to this chakra and so it will be important to notice any breathing issues that may be present while you are going through healing in this area.

Mental

Thoughts of love, community, and friendship are the reality of the heart chakra. Most people will only think with their heads and not carefully weigh in on what the heart wants. It can be a harder journey to opening the chakras if you don't let your heart have a say in the matter. Your heart is actually not only made of cardiovascular cells and tissues but neurons as well. Neurons are brain cells. Your heart has the capacity to think, not just feel.

If you are imbalanced in the heart chakra your thoughts may not be very open-hearted and you may tend to express yourself selfishly and indifferently to other people.

Emotional

Emotions are often either overactive, underactive, or stagnant within the chakras. The stagnant or blocked heart chakra isn't able to openly love or let love in. There will be issues of loving others excessively and for selfish reasons, suffocating the person or people (overactive), or there will be a total denial of affection and coldness when it comes to loving others.

This chakra is also about the feelings and emotions surround self-love and a lot of times this chakra can get blocked when we are not able to love ourselves unconditionally.

Spiritual

Spiritually, the heart chakra is all about unity consciousness and brotherly love. It has to do with feeling warm and open to your fellow man and woman, no matter their age, race, or background. When this chakra is blocked there can be issues of collective judgment, ridicule, racism, and so forth.

The balancing of this chakra is an important step in opening all of the others because it helps you radiate energy at a higher frequency, allowing you to help your other chakras by feeling the love vibration for yourself, and those around you.

5. <u>**The Throat Chakra**</u>

Physical

The thyroid gland, which produces several hormones, is responsible for growth, metabolism, and regulating body temperature. This gland is situated in the neck in the area of the larynx and vocal cords. Physical imbalances that arise here include thyroid problems (hypo/hyperactive), throat, neck, teeth and jaw problems, vocal nodes, and any issues related to throat.

There are also lung-related issues associated with this chakra, including asthma, bronchitis, or chronic congestion. Even though the lungs are also connected to the heart chakra, it is mostly the throat chakra imbalances that demonstrate respiratory issues.

Mental

This chakra deals with the issue of communication in all its forms, including speech, writing, and sound. Here is where expressions of thought are verbally expressed and so if you have a blocked or imbalanced throat, you may have issues with communicating your thoughts. That could mean overcommunicating them, or not communicating them at all.

You may find that with the throat chakra in excess you will be more inclined to talk constantly without much of an ability to other people's thoughts or ideas. Additionally, deficient energy here will make it feel impossible for you to share your ideas, or speak your opinions. That can lead to being considered under or over-opinionated.

Emotional

Emotionally, you may feel shy, unheard, afraid to share, and like your opinions and ideas don't matter. The feelings related to this chakra have a tendency to make it hard for people to be themselves which links to the solar plexus, or that there is a blocked ability to creatively express the self, linking to the sacral chakra.

Spiritual

On a spiritual level, the throat chakra is the voice of truth and if it is open and balanced, you have a very clear way of speaking your own truth. This can also lead to being able to hear and respond to the Universe more openly. Talking to "source" comes from this chakra, and you can be sure that a lot of people pray out loud sometimes. Prayer isn't really what it's about, though. It's about communication with something bigger than you. A blocked throat makes this impossible.

6. <u>The Brow (Third Eye) Chakra</u>

Physical

Your pituitary gland is linked to your third eye and is responsible for the release of hormones into your bloodstream. It relates to growth and has an important function to help other glands in the endocrine system function properly. The pineal gland is also affiliated with this chakra, being so close in location to the forehead.

Issues with the eyes, like glaucoma, arise when this chakra is imbalanced. It relates to neurological issues and disorders, headaches and migraines, and most things related to the brain, skull and central nervous system.

Mental

A deficiency in positive energy flow here leads to rigid thinking and relying on other people's ideas and beliefs, rather than thinking for yourself. It is also possible to have an excess of energy here which will lead to delusions and, worst-case scenario, hallucinations, and fantastical thinking. You might also just appear a little too heady, always lost in the clouds and not really paying much attention to the important things on the ground.

Emotional

On an emotional level, the third eye asks you to be very open to a lot of different ideas and your relationship to the Universe and everything around you in new ways. This can be a little terrifying and the result of imbalance here can lead to a lot of paranoia, anxiety, worry, fear, disbelief, and insomnia.

There are a lot of ways that these emotional patterns get thought of as mental illness, or something requiring excessive therapy or even medication when really there is a need to balance the energy.

Spiritual

This is the place of your psychic power and clairvoyance. It is a much greater and deeper connection to all things in the Universe. It is also a way for you to learn how to live your life as a totally open person who has gained true knowledge of self and spirit. This is where wisdom is of value and a lot of people take it too far and develop an egotistical and prideful mind state that overrides the wisdom of the third eye.

7. <u>**The Crown Chakra**</u>

Physical

The pineal gland is connected to the crown chakra (and also the third eye) and regulates body rhythms, specifically sleep through the secretion of melatonin. An issue here might mean an issue with sleep. This chakra is closely linked to the third eye, as they are such close neighbors, and so they will sometimes have similar physical imbalances.

The crown connects to issues with the central nervous system, spinal cord, brain stem and all of your nerves and pain centers. Epilepsy is often affiliated with this chakra, as well as other seizure-type disorders.

Mental

The mental imbalances of this chakra are a lot like the third eye and deal with the aspect of being over-intellectual and pragmatic about information. There are ways that the mind will only see one thing one way and will demonstrate rigidity of thought. There can also be an attitude of prejudice or criticism.

Mental imbalances here could also lead to dementia, schizophrenia and other psychotic disorders that may be misdiagnosed as being only clinical and physical and not related to energy imbalances or blockages.

Emotional

Emotionally, this is where you would feel the world coming down on you all at once. It can feel scary, suffocating, too big, and difficult to process. This is where most people feel the emotions of an 'existential crisis.' It can feel like you are so incredibly alone and like there will never be anyone who can possibly understand what it is like for you.

The emotions of this chakra are closely linked to the reality of becoming enlightened and all of the purging that is required to exist in a transcendent state of mind. This can be what the imbalances are directly related to so that it appears as mental illness or instability of mind, when it is actually a rebalancing and reconfiguring of your beliefs to make room for enlightened thought and emotion.

Spiritual

This chakra is the seat of enlightenment and it correlates to spiritual wisdom, truth, oneness, dynamic thought. This is the spiritual center and if you have an imbalance here you are totally disconnected from your deeper wisdom and spiritual truth. There are a lot of gurus out there, trying to show people, lead them, or make them see, but no one can do that for you.

Following the advice of gurus can be seen as an imbalance of the crown chakra because until you seek that truth, wisdom, and knowledge on your own, you cannot become enlightened.

The physical, mental, emotional, and spiritual imbalances of each of the chakras are never definite. You should always consult your doctor if you are suffering from any serious illness, especially if you need regular medical attention.

In addition to working with your regular health care and wellness plan, understanding how the chakras affect each one of these systems will help you recognize where you can begin to heal yourself. You may want to start with a certain chakra because it relates to your glandular problem or your chronic fatigue syndrome.

Once you begin to heal one chakra you will quickly find how closely related to each other they can be and how these connections are a beautiful and intricate internal puzzle of energy. You get to be your very own energy detective and solve the mystery of where you are out of balance and how to get started with purging, clearing and cleansing all of these imbalances. Once you get going, it just keeps going.

Now that you have all of this knowledge about your chakras, it is time to examine them. The next chapter will offer you a series of questions that you can start to ask to help you determine the health of your chakras.

Chapter 7: Examining Your Chakras: Questions to Ask on Your Healing Path

The chakra healing path is a very personal experience and it begins with your ability to ask yourself some important questions. When you are in greater awareness of your true feelings, you can begin to honor how to make changes to the parts of your life that need transformation. Awareness is the first step to healing yourself.

In this chapter, you will be guided through a series of questions to help you understand where *you* stand in your energy system. Each set of questions will correspond with each of the seven chakras to help you ascertain the quality of each part of the system. Keep in mind while you are answering these questions that it is never just one chakra that is off-balance. Usually, if there is one that is having notable issues, the core problem may be coming from another chakra.

An example of this could be feeling like you are not very open to receiving love and have a hard time loving yourself. You immediately assume that the main cause of this corresponds to a blocked heart chakra. What you may not recognize right away is that your heart chakra issues are more deeply rooted in your base chakra, the root, where you are holding onto childhood pain from feeling unloved by your family? Get the picture?

To help heal your chakras, you get to play the role of personal detective and try to connect some dots. It may not be obvious at first, but the more you ask questions about how you are feeling in each center, the more answers you will find, and the more of the "You Puzzle" you will actually see.

Take your time answering these questions. You can also refer back to them at any point during your healing experience and notice what changes have occurred along the way. The way you answer a question today will likely be a very different answer in a few months or even weeks from now.

The Root Chakra Questions:

1. Do you have issues bringing money into your household?

2. Do you feel like you are unable to allow anyone to get to close to you?

3. Are you able to trust anyone you meet, or do you tend to distrust immediately and warily build trust over time?

4. Do you have a lot of issues with your family members, like parents, siblings, or early caregivers?

5. Do you have severe aches, tension, tightness, or pain in any of the following: hips, low back, knees, ankles, or feet?

6. Are you involved in anything that forces you to act in a constant state of survival, for example, drug and alcohol addiction, crime, unhealthy or abusive relationships, or serious debt?

7. Would you consider yourself a stickler for savings and are you always thinking about money and where to put it, influence it, make it, or save it?

8. Are you able to let others share your wealth, or are you more controlling with your abundance?

9. Do you feel like you have everything that you need (not want, but need) in your life right now?

10. Do you feel secure in your home, family, finances, and health?

A balanced root chakra allows you to feel grounded and secure within your home, family, career, and financial assets. You will also have the capacity to give and share your wealth and will not express greed or stinginess. You will feel stable on your legs and feet and will have a fluidity of movement in your lower body. Your energy will be in good condition because your adrenal cortex will be in good, working condition. You won't have to work so hard to survive because all of your needs will feel met.

After answering these questions, review what you are feeling about what your responses were. You will notice right away if there are imbalances here that need some chakra healing therapy. You can apply this practice to every set of questions that follow.

You can also start a notebook or journal to ask these questions and come back to them in a couple of months and see if your answers will be the same. Sometimes, tracking your progress can feel very motivating, especially when you are able to notice real changes in how you are feeling or answering these important questions.

The Sacral Chakra Questions:

1. Are you physically open to other people, or are you able to respond to intimacy with other people?

2. Do you feel an urge to have sex or to pleasure yourself on a regular basis?

3. Are you able to work with creative tools without fear, like paint, paper and pen, drawing, sculpting, and other crafts?

4. Do you spend time singing and dancing?

5. Are you afraid to connect to others sexually, or do you have a lot of fear of your own sexuality, even when you are alone?

6. Have you attempted to start a family, but have had issues conceiving?

7. Are you able to have regular menstruation (if you are a woman), or are you able to regularly ejaculate (if you are a man)?

8. Do you feel disconnected from your body?

9. Do you feel creatively blocked, like you can't get anything done the way you want it to look, feel, taste, sound, etc.?

10. Do you live your life with passion and verve, or are you a bit more stoic and aloof?

A balanced sacral chakra will allow you to feel present with your body and able to share your intimate self with another. You will be able to enjoy a healthy sex-life and have an openness about connecting with others on this level. You will enjoy your passionate nature without being overly emotional. You can have a more creative experience as well. This doesn't mean that you have to be an artist, but rather that your ability to live life in a creative attitude is expanded. You will feel balanced in your reproductive organs and your cycles, as well as having healthy secretions of hormones so that you are feeling healthy in all of these areas.

The Solar Plexus Chakra Questions:

1. Are you confident in who you are as a person?

2. When other people have great ideas to share, do you feel like you have to one-up them somehow to be the better, more interesting person?

3. Would you be more likely to shy away when someone else or a group of people want to know more about you?

4. Do you have any issues with your digestion or ability to process certain foods?

5. Is your blood sugar a concern for you?

6. Would you call yourself a dominant or a submissive person, or are you somewhere in the middle?

7. Are you accepting of your abilities, skills, talents, and gifts that you can offer to the world?

8. Do you usually feel exhausted, or do you have a lot of energy that you don't always know what to do with?

9. Are you able to ask others for what you want and need, or are you afraid to bother anyone with your needs?

10. Are you happy with who you are and what you are doing with your life?

A Balanced solar plexus chakra allows you to feel confident in what you like, feel, believe, enjoy, and how you are expressing yourself to the world. You are able to feel energetic and empowered on a regular basis and feel attractive on all levels. You are not domineering, nor are you shy; you are grounded in your identity and work well with others as a result. You are likely to enjoy a variety of foods without any serious digestive, or insulin issues and have a lot of energy for healthy exercise and stamina for all kinds of life adventures.

The Heart Chakra Questions:

1. Are you open to another person's offering of love or do you try to push it away?

2. Do you feel like it is easy for you to feel compassion for other people or are you more likely to judge first and act compassionately later?

3. What are your feelings about other people from other races, cultures, and religions? Are you open-hearted, interested and loving or are you biased, critical, and judgemental?

4. Do you suffer from any known heart conditions?

5. Do you have circulation issues, edema, varicose veins, high or low blood pressure, or any other heart or circulation issue?

6. Is there anyone in your life that makes you feel truly happy and loved?

7. Are you able to fully love yourself, without conditions, rules, flaws and all, and without criticism or judgment?

8. Do you cling to others out of fear of losing their love?

9. Do you offer love to others for selfish reasons, as in having an expectation that they will give you as much or more in return?

10. Are you asking yourself if you have what you want or if you have what makes you happy on a regular basis?

A balanced heart chakra will allow you to feel love in all its forms. It isn't just about romantic love for a partner; it's also about how we give love to friends, family, neighbors, strangers, and other groups, cultures, and races. When you are healthy in this chakra you are able to love yourself and others easily without any need of anything in return for your love. You will have a healthy heart and circulation throughout the body and will also have an ability to take clear, deep, long breaths. You can feel attached to others without needing them to love you back and you can offer your compassion and love in return without expecting the same.

The Throat Chakra Questions:

1. Is your voice available to you to speak freely and often about what matters to you?

2. Are you able to listen well to others and give space for others to talk about themselves and their opinions?

3. Is it a struggle for you to talk about yourself or be expressive in a group situation?

4. Do you have any regularly occurring ear, nose, or throat issues, like infections, drainage, stuffy nose, congestion, sore throat, etc.?

5. Are you avoiding saying what you actually want to a lot of the time?

6. Has anyone ever told you that you talk too much and they can never get a word in edgewise?

7. Are you able to consistently tell the truth or do you find yourself telling little white lies all of the time?

8. Do you have a history of lung issues, or do you smoke a lot of cigarettes?

9. Are you afraid to hear what another person might say about you, yet you are freely saying similar things to others?

10. Are you able to express your true feelings in the moment or when it is necessary?

An open throat chakra allows you to communicate with ease and calm. You can express your truth and have no reason or cause to lie about anything. In addition, you are able to allow others to say what they need to say and act as a good listener, instead of only talking about yourself and your beliefs. You are able to creatively express yourself through speech, writing, and sound and are able to let go of any issues around the need to say what you feel and think. You will have healthier sinuses and lungs and will be able to draw breath through your mouth and nose very easily.

The Brow (Third Eye) Chakra Questions:

1. Are you a visual person, or is it hard for you to picture things in your mind's eye?

2. Do you have an overactive imagination to the point where you live in a fantasy or daydream world?

3. Do you suffer from paranoia, unreasonable fears, and doubts, or anxiety about life or what's to come?

4. Do you trust your intuition?

5. Are you able to allow for your inner noise to quiet and allow for a clear mind space?

6. Do you believe in the possibility of angels, spirit guides, or dimensions out of your realm of understanding?

7. Do you have psychic dreams or visions, or do you disbelieve that you are actually capable of them?

8. Are you in alignment with your true purpose or are you uncertain of what that purpose is?

9. Is there a place in your head that makes you feel like you are insane or unstable because of some of the ways that you think about life?

10. Do you suffer from mental health issues that require therapy or medication?

A balanced third eye chakra allows you to explore reality in new ways and will also show you how to manifest your true life purpose through being 'awakened' to your spiritual self. You will have more understanding about the way the Universe works and will be more likely to connect to your psychic abilities, clairvoyance, and spiritual guidance. You will have a grounded attitude about being connected to more than just the Earth and will likely feel like you are a bigger part of a greater whole. You will have a calm attitude and a wise approach to making your reality the truest for you.

The Crown Chakra Questions:

1. Do you feel like answers to common questions just don't make sense anymore?

2. Do you feel like an outcast, living on the fringe because you aren't quite sure where you fit in anymore?

3. Are you uncomfortable in accepting what the news says is a reality?

4. Are you an adamant conspiracy theorist about almost everything?

5. Do you look at others and feel like they are all idiotic and repressed and that there is no hope for humanity?

6. Do you desire to learn more than what you were taught by family, school, culture, and society because you just know there is something more?

7. Do you suffer from headaches, delusions, dementia, eye issues, or trouble sleeping?

8. Are you asking yourself if you are really here
   or if this is just a simulation program you are
   going to experience before your next 'life'?

9. Do you feel like you don't have control over
   any of your choices?

10. Are you indifferent to the bigger questions?

A balanced crown chakra allows you to feel enlightened and awakened to your true spiritual wisdom and personal authority. When you are aligned in this chakra you are more likely to feel at peace with the nature of humanity and the cosmos. You will always feel like you are wanted and that you belong and that you are unique energy that is important to the flow of all energy in the world. You will feel a balance in all of your other chakra centers and will have a better grasp on why we are all here and that we are evolving as we are meant to.

Spend time with these questions and revisit them as often as you need to so that you can measure your chakra awakening progress. Your answers are likely to change if you are doing the healing work and each set of questions will help you see where you need the most healing right now. It's a great place to get you started. In the next chapter, you will discover more of the benefits of healing the chakras and why it will be an excellent way for you to feel the balance, harmony, peace, and well-being that you deserve.

Chapter 8: Chakra Healing Benefits

You have probably already noticed how beneficial it can be to heal your chakras from what you have already read in this book. There are so many amazing applications for this kind of energy care and maintenance and as you go forward on your healing path you will discover so much more about how it actually feels to operate on higher levels of health and well-being.

You cannot imagine what it feels like, especially if you have never tried this kind of healing and awakening journey and so the best way there is to just start implementing it into your regular routines and rituals for health care. You can easily see from the chapter on imbalances and the previous chapter full of questions that there are so many different layers to healing the chakras. This chapter will go over more of the benefits from the different levels of the self again: physical, mental, emotional, and spiritual.

Physical Benefits

- Improved energy, stamina, and general feelings of wellness

- Endocrine system functioning optimally allowing for healthy and responsive hormone secretions

- Fewer regular illness

- Relief of chronic problems over time

- Regression of cancer, in some cases

- Healing benefits during chemotherapy

- Healing of diabetic problems, in some cases

- Relief of symptoms caused by allergies, common colds, cases of flu, etc.

- Calming effects before, during, and after surgery

- Healing of certain chronic fatigue disorders and diseases

- Feelings of tension, achiness, soreness, and stiffness released and healed

- A general feeling of being fitter and freer in range of motion

- Symptoms related to digestive disorders and diseases are balanced and cured, in some cases

- Relief of migraines and headaches

- An overall feeling of relaxation and inner calm and peace

Mental Benefits

- Soothing effects that leave you feeling clear of mind and at peace with thoughts

- General ability to think clearly and have improved cognitive abilities

- Improved memory

- Healing of certain neurological disorders, in some cases

- A general shift in some mental health issues, including dementia, schizophrenia, and paranoia

- Sense of well-being allowing for a higher mind function

- Clearly expressed thoughts and ideas through healthy communication

- A shift in beliefs, values, and attitudes

- Thought patterns altered for good, as in the change in habits that are unhealthy

- Healthier thoughts about self and others

- Fewer limiting beliefs

- Acceptance of the words, opinions, thoughts, and expressions of others

- Clairvoyance and psychic understanding

- Higher wisdom

- Capacity to understand humanity and the Universe in bigger, broader ways

Emotional Benefits

- Lack of fear or anxiety about life matters

- Feelings of security and groundedness

- Ability to give and receive love in healthy, balanced ways

- Acceptance of flaws and allowance of true self-expression

- Partnerships that are healthy, meaningful, and stable

- Passion, desire, and creative attitude toward life

- Sexually open, healthy, and balanced with other parts of the self

- Emotionally agile and flexible without getting overwrought and intense about any situation

- Calm, serene, and grounded behaviors, overall

- Lack of guilt, shame, doubt, or self-repression

- Feelings of joy, ebullience, progressiveness, and happiness in life

- Open-hearted to all cultures, race, and backgrounds

- Feelings of love for all mankind and the Universe as a whole

- Affection and love for the self on all levels

- Balance with all relationships and feelings involved in them

- Expressiveness from both the heart and the mind and not just one or the other

Spiritual Benefits

- Opening to the higher mind and higher self

- Spiritual wisdom

- Opening of the third eye, psychic abilities, clairvoyance, and claircognizance

- Powerful connection to deeper truth and purpose in this life

- Expansion of beliefs, values, and ideals

- Comradery with all other people

- Determination to keep 'knowing' and seeking answers to the bigger, deeper questions

- Feelings of joy and abundance all of the time

- Connection to a God-like source, or creation energy

- Feelings of never needing anything; that you already are and have everything you need

- Enlightenment

- Powerful experiences with energy, vibrations, and frequencies that can be felt in the body

- Kundalini Awakening

- Chakra balancing and wholeness

No matter what your purposes are for healing your chakras and balancing your internal energy, the benefits are powerful and are a true reality for many people who have started the healing path and seen magnificent change, transformation, and overall feelings of lightness and joy.

There are so many different ways that these benefits will manifest in your life and as you will see as you continue to read, the journey has only just begun. The next several chapters will give more instruction about how to heal the chakras now that you are better acquainted with them. Prepare for your healing journey and let the benefits speak for themselves.

Chapter 9: How to Heal Your Chakras

When you are ready to start working on awakening the chakras, there are a variety of ways that you can take charge of this healing by yourself and also with the assistance and help of other sources. Some of the methods in this chapter will be discussed in greater detail in later chapters, so this is more of an overview of methods and techniques to get you started.

The variations of these techniques are dependent upon you, your preferences, and where you are going to seek additional help. There are some tools that are best handled by people who are trained in their skill, but you can actually learn many of these skills and take all of your healing into your own hands.

Starting off with your first ideas for healing, you can begin to shift a lot of your energy by going to see some different specialists who can begin to help you unblock your energies on a deep level. The next section will give you more specifics about what I mean.

How to Heal Your Chakras with Assistance

There are several different approaches to healing the chakras through variations of alternative medicine and energy healing practices. These techniques are simple, affordable, and are widely available in most places.

Yoga

Yoga is a widely practiced form of body movement and breathing techniques that is actually from the same culture that originally described the chakras in their ancient, religious texts. Yoga is specifically designed to balance your energy and keep you in a healthy frame of mind, flexibility of body, and lightness of spirit.

All of the various forms of yoga incorporate specific poses that are structures to allow certain parts of your body to heal, depending on what you are trying to accomplish. There are also different styles of breathing techniques that complement the yoga poses, or asanas so that you are bringing healthy doses of oxygen to your muscles, joints, and organ systems.

This body practice is not just for physical health, it is also for your mental and spiritual well-being and many people practice it over other kinds of exercise because of the long list of health benefits. From the perspective of healing and awakening the chakras, it happens to be one of the best forms of exercise and physical training you can do.

There is even a specific kind of yoga that was created for the purpose of awakening your kundalini, the dormant life force that lives in the base of your spine in the root chakra. This kind of yoga is meant to spark that awakening and heal the chakras through movement, postures and breathing techniques. It is specifically called Kundalini Yoga.

You can most likely sign up for any yoga class, or a Kundalini class, in your area as soon as you are ready. There are usually a lot of options and places to practice and once you learn the general postures and breaths, you can begin to do all of these exercises on your own at home.

In fact, many people today are using online yoga classes to have a free, everyday routine to keep them going. It can be as easy as opening up your phone or computer first thing in the morning and making it a part of your regular routine.

Yoga is always a good choice for this kind of healing work. Try a variety of styles and decide which one works best for you right now. You can try each of them at different times in your awakening as they are all very different and will a different impact on your overall energy.

Acupuncture

Acupuncture is also a well-known alternative medicine that is a part of Traditional Chinese Medicine and has made its way across the world to a variety of cultures in the West. In Traditional Chinese Medicine, the chakra energy is referred to as Chi and is said to flow through what are called meridians in the body. These meridians are basically a system of channels that this life-force energy flows through and there are a variety of practices in China that are used to help benefit the flow of Chi.

Tai chi is considered a martial art and has been used to keep a balance of the flow of the energy within, just as acupuncture is meant to do. For this practice, there are points all over the body where needles are placed to stimulate energy flow and rebalancing. These points are considered to be tiny chakras and can be influenced by the prick of a needle.

Whatever you are ailing from, acupuncture points will stimulate change in your system to help those ailments find a better flow of energy to support healing and recovery, even when all you are looking for is peace of mind and relaxation.

Acupuncture is available in a wide variety of clinics all over the world and sometimes you can find them in spaces where other healing services are performed, like Reiki and massage. Either one of these would be excellent additions to your ongoing chakra healing therapy, especially Reiki which brings us to the next section:

Reiki

Reiki is designed to heal the chakras. It is based on the ancient wisdom of the Hindu religions and was developed by a Buddhist monk who was studying the writings of Buddha and methods for healing and enlightenment. He was born in Japan and so the name for the practice is a Japanese word, but the practice is universal.

Reiki practitioners and Masters are attuned to act as a channel for healing and are able to influence the chakras through their own energetic ability to heal these centers through touch, or by hovering over the chakras and connecting to that energy. The possibilities with healing through Reiki are endless.

Many people have discovered this miraculous treatment and have even become practitioners after experiencing it. A client will lie on a massage table and the Reiki practitioner will work with their auras and chakras to pull out unwanted or stagnant energies, unblocking each area and making more space for better energy flow and more opportunity for healing.

The chakras are easily affected by this kind of treatment and although the results can fluctuate between being very obvious and very subtle, the energy transformation cannot be mistaken.

You are likely to find several Reiki Masters and practitioners in your local community. Working with this kind of healer is a great way to do some awakening work and if you like the results, you can actually take classes to do reiki on yourself. It is the first thing you learn to do in a Reiki attunement: self-healing. Self-healing is the ultimate goal and although it would be nice to take care of every single need we have, sometimes we need help from others

The next section will talk more about ways you can heal your chakras on your own.

How to Heal Your Chakras on Your Own

All of the above methods work well in addition to what you can do on your own time at home. The practice of healing the self requires consistency and devotion. I trust you are already capable of knowing that it is in your hands and that you get to decide how much and how often, but if you are really hoping to inspire change, everyday practice on some level is ideal.

Mantras

Mantras are an amazingly powerful tool. They are simple sounds, words, or phrases that elicit a specific internal and external consequence. There are a lot of mantras out there and it can be confusing to decide what mantras work best for which situations. Fortunately, Chapter 11 is all about the mantras you need to successfully maintain chakra health and balance.

The point of mantras is to inform the mind of what you want. Thoughts can be very hurtful, accusatory, and demeaning to who you are and what you want. The idea of the mantra is to rephrase the thoughts that are keeping you down or low so that your mind forms newer, more emotionally intelligent neural pathways to think on.

A mantra doesn't have to be a specific word or phrase to have meaning. Have you ever heard of the classic word, 'Om'? Om is used quite regularly in yoga practices and other meditative experiences and it helps you to connect to deeper energy within your body, and it is also a mantra.

Mantras are energy and as you will discover later, they are an excellent way to transform your energy from negative to positive and to keep your chakras in a good balance.

Meditations

Meditation is no new thing. It is one of the hottest buzz words, still. The work you do around meditation is a lot simpler than many people might think. The basics are that you sit in stillness, clear your mind, and enter a present state with yourself. This is not as easy as it sounds because we have a lot of thoughts, feelings, worries, and so forth that make it hard to stay centered and focus only on the emptiness in the mind.

It takes a little practice, but a few minutes a day of quiet reflection and solitude works wonders, no matter what thoughts might be floating through the cloud space in your mind. There are a lot more tips, pointers and steps for you in Chapter 12 so that you can actually start your own guided meditations today.

When you take the time to meditate, you are taking the time to connect to your energy and then make it possible to hear it, understand what is going on in your life, and clear anything that is causing you problems or difficulties.

Crystals

Crystals are strong, energetic objects. They are made by the Earth and they carry positive healing vibrations and higher frequencies. There are so many different varieties and colors and each has a different purpose and meaning. You can find hundreds and hundreds of them and learn as much as you want about the power of each gemstone or crystal.

Chapter 13 will give you some more specifics and offer some healing opportunities to explore these tools. You can actually place them over any one of your chakras and let it sit there for 10-30 minutes while you close your eyes and meditate. The energy of the crystal connects with the energy of the chakra and from there will help to purge, balance and transmute the energy of that placement.

There are even specific stones for a specific chakra. The crystals will usually share the qualities of the chakra so that when you are applying that crystal to the chakra it connects to, you are informing that chakra of how it wants to feel through the energy of the stone.

Exploring crystals will help you find what you need to expedite the transformation process. Crystals are like putting a magnifying glass on the issue and burning it out with light, as is the case with Reiki on the chakras.

Reiki and Yoga

As you have already learned, Reiki is a healing method that has evolved from ancient wisdom and techniques. It is often applied through service with someone known as a practitioner or a Master who has a higher degree of Reiki training. One thing you can actually do to help your healing journey is to get trained to do Reiki on yourself.

The techniques are divided into three levels of learning and the first level is for students who are only interested in practicing this healing technique on their own bodies. It can be a very helpful and powerful method for healing quickly and you can find a Reiki Master to give you the lessons in your local community. You may have to pay for the class and it will likely take the length of a weekend workshop, but after that, you will have another excellent tool to heal yourself with.

Yoga is also something you can teach yourself and inventing your own daily routine or yoga ritual will provide you with ongoing healing of the chakra energy and keeping it a good balance. There are even yoga poses that are specific to each chakra so if you feel like you are out of balance in one area or chakra, you can design a yoga practice that will be specific to the needs of that chakra.

Either, or both, of these practices, would be an excellent addition to working with meditations, mantras, and crystals. The more you do, the faster you heal.

Additional Tips, Hints, and Ideas

This section will provide some additional bullet points of things that will definitely work to help you heal your chakras, on more than one level:

- Spend time in nature, hiking, walking, lying in the grass, gardening, or anything else that you like to do outdoors.

- Dance, dance, dance, like nobody, is watching.

- Play a musical instrument, even if you think you are terrible and have no skill. The point is to make sound, not to be a pop star.

- Eat well. This means fresh vegetables, fruits, nuts, and lean meats with lots of water and low intake of alcohol, sugar, caffeine, and processed foods with ingredients you can't pronounce the names of easily.

- Hobbies. Find your hobbies and passions and make them a part of your life.

- Listen to music, any kind of music.

- Take time to go to places you have never been to before, even if it is in your hometown or city.

- Look at art, in museums, in books, or online.

- Get involved in some kind of community service.

- Take a class you have always wanted to take. Expand your knowledge.

- Design your daily life to include only what you want to do, not just what you feel like you have to, even when it means working a lot.

- Share your stories and experiences with other people.

- Try something you have always been afraid of.

- Practice with your intuition and see how well you already know what you think you don't.

- Sleep and rest well.

All of these tips and pointers seem like common sense, but all too often each of us forgets what we can do to improve our energy and our health. These activities are actually helpful ways to alter your chakra energy for the better. When you give your energy what it actually wants and needs, you are offering yourself healing and balance.

All of these possibilities work well together, or slowly and separately over time. You don't have to do everything all at once. Whatever is standing out the most to you right now is probably the best place to start. Use your intuition. The next chapter will briefly discuss ways that other people can influence your energy and helpful ways that you can stay grounded and free of negative energy in these situations.

Chapter 10: How Other People Affect Your Chakras

If you have learned anything so far it is that we are all energy and we all have a chakra system. Our chakras play a huge role in the quality of our feelings, personality, general health and well-being, and the way we openly express ourselves to others. In many cases, people are not thinking about the ways their energy is affecting anyone else's, but we are all most definitely aware when someone's negative attitude bothers us.

The way we input or interpret when someone else has "bad" or poor energy is to either feel it through our own energy or block it through effort so that we don't take it on and make it a part of us. Allow me to explain more of how this works:

Your chakras are the 7 energy centers in your body, all of them connected to specific thoughts, emotions, and so forth. Your auras are an extension of that energy and are layered from the skin to about 18 inches outside of your body, or more! The root chakra aura is closest to the skin and the crown chakra aura is the farthest from your body, behaving like an antenna to receive "energetic input".

This is how people can sense when a storm is coming or that they just walked into a room where someone had a fight just moments before. Our antennas are our chakras and auras combined and they are always sensing the world around you. Without even realizing you are doing it you are picking up on everyone and everything. It may not be a very intense signal and you may not feel the effects of that energy while you sit in your chair and read your book, sipping your hot coffee, but the energy is there with you.

Let's say you are having an amazing morning with your kids and you have a great meal before setting off to work, feeling uplifted and excited for life. As you walk into your office, you suddenly feel gloomy and you might think to yourself, "Ugh, I don't want to be here," or you might recognize after a few minutes of information gathering that several people are getting laid off and so the air in the room is anxious and uncomfortable.

The energy of each of us can connect and collectively make an impact, as with the example of the office above. It doesn't even have to be a whole group of people to have an impact either. You could be minding your own business, having a lovely day, when some curmudgeonly person scowls at you, offended that you dared to smile and enjoy yourself. That energy radiating off of another person and directed at you is enough to shift your chakras and your thoughts and feelings along with them. You might even pick up that sour feeling from that individual, unable to shake it for the rest of the day.

The reason we are all so affected by each other is that we all have our own imbalances and chakra mysteries to solve and it can be a real challenge to identify that at the moment, keeping yourself positive and grounded without feeling the effects of someone else's energy.

You can easily remove unwanted energies that you collect from other people through your chakra cleansing and balancing techniques and routines and you can also protect yourself ahead of time with the same techniques. The term 'grounding' is used frequently when people are talking about their energy and it makes sense!

If you think about electricity, which is a form of energy, oftentimes electrical inputs and outputs are connected to what is called a 'grounding wire'. This wire runs from an electrical box to the ground so that the current of electricity has another place to safely travel in the event of a short circuit.

Now think of that in terms of people and their energy currents. You are the electrical box and the grounding wire is your tool to stay connected to yourself and no one else's energy. A short circuit might be an emotional outburst directed at you or someone's sour attitude that has nothing to do with you. The point of grounding is that you are stabilizing yourself so that you are not as likely to be affected by other people's energy.

Sometimes the question will arise, "but, what if I am helping someone who is sad or in pain, and I feel compassion for them, and feel their sadness and pain, too?"

The emotion of compassion is an important energy to resonate towards another, and you can express compassion without actually taking on the pain of another. This will also require grounding. It is important as you go through healing and awakening your chakras that you can tell the difference between your feelings and someone else's.

What do you ask yourself when you are in these situations? Do you even have time to think or do you just react? What are some of the ways you already know you pick up other people's energy in your everyday life? Are there perhaps one or two individuals who are especially energetically intense in your life? Are you able to put yourself into a different connection to them so that you don't accept their energy and make it your own?

There are so many possible ways that you can pick up on the energy of anyone around you and having a good presence with your own energy by staying grounded is a good skill to have while you work on your healing process. The next section will give you some pointers and tips on how to ground your energy so that you are able to handle whatever comes your way.

Steps to Grounding Yourself

All of the skills that you will learn in the next few chapters will be of use to you in helping you stay grounded. The main tools you will learn for healing your chakras involve mantras, meditations, and crystals. Each of these tools could be used separately or together as a way to ground your energy and so as you continue learning these skills you can bring them forward for healing, balancing and grounding.

1. Before you go out into the world, to run errands or head to work, take a few minutes in the morning to connect to your energy.

2. Close your eyes and take some deep breaths. Think about possible ways that you might be affected by other energies: careless or aggressive drivers, challenging co-workers who talk your ear off, rush hour traffic.

3. Consider what your normal reaction to these situations, or people might be and assign some words or thoughts to them: frustrated, annoyed, angry, bitter, concerned, anxious.

4. Think about how strong those energies are and how they affect you. They aren't really

about you at all and they are coming from other people's feelings about life.

5. Meditate on what feelings you would prefer to feel in these moments: relaxed, calm, serene, understanding, positive, kind, generous, protected, unphased.

6. Come up with a mantra or affirmation that will help you at any moment that you feel might be challenging. It could actually be any word that will remind you to put your energy back toward you and ground it with that word. An example word might be "focus" or "breathe". You could also say something like, "It's not you. I am here." Whatever the mantra is, say it in those moments that are affecting your energy in a negative way.

7. Take a few more deep breaths and move forward in your day.

8. Use your mantra throughout the course of your day and add the following tip...

Another way you can ground yourself is to carry a crystal or gemstone that has grounding energy. You will learn more about these stones in Chapter 13 and the good thing is that you can find them in a variety of sizes so they are easy to carry with you in your pocket. Having a grounding stone will connect to your chakra energy and auras always assisting and aiding you.

If you are feeling really affected by someone or something you can hold it in the palm of your hand or rub it between your fingers to help you connect to it more effectively.

All of these tools will bring you into a more grounded focus so that you can be ready to handle anyone's energy, no matter the situation. Taking deep breaths, meditating, using a mantra, and carrying a grounding stone will keep you feeling awareness about your energy and that you don't have to absorb anyone else's.

The next chapter will get you started with more mantras and some of the best ones you can use to maintain chakra health and balance.

Chapter 11: Chakra Mantras: 20 of the Most Beneficial Mantras for Maintaining Chakra Health

What is a mantra? Mantras have been used for centuries all over the world in a variety of methods, languages, and for various purposes. They are very simple tools that have a powerful energetic impact on your whole being and will carry you forward in your life on new levels of happiness, joy, and health.

The basic mantras that you will come across in a lot of yoga practices or meditation rituals are simply one word that is intoned through a long breath out. You certainly don't have to enjoy a mantra out loud like this; you can also just repeat it in your head as many times as you want to get the point across.

Mantras are a timeless tool and amazingly enough, there are mantras that are specifically coordinated to each of your seven chakras. As you engage with these mantras you can ask yourself what is wanted from that energy. The words that you use will resonate with that chakra and will have an effect on that energy.

If you focus your mind on that chakra center as you are saying in your mind or out loud what the mantra is, you will be asking that energy become more awakened, opened and balanced. These 7 mantras listed below are just the beginning of what you can do with a healing word.

The Root Chakra: LAAM (lahm)

This word, LAAM, is the energy clearing and cleansing word for the root chakra. It will help to keep you grounded and rooted in the energy of the earth. You can chant this mantra several times and as you do it will help to release blockages of energy and impurities that have collected in this energy center.

The word will open you up to the feelings of the healthy and balanced root chakra, such as the sense of belonging, security, stability, abundance, and prosperity. It will also help to clear the path for other chakras to flow well with the main root.

If you are feeling any of the root chakra imbalances you have learned about, chant or intone aloud, or say in your mind several times while you picture your red root swirling freely and openly.

The Sacral Chakra: VAAM (vahm)

This mantra taps into the energy of your creativity, passion, sexuality, and pleasure. You can chant or intone this mantra aloud, or say it in your mind. It is typically more powerful to say it out loud if you are in a space where you are comfortable doing that.

Having an opening in this energy center allows you to express yourself creatively and well, and helps you open yourself to others easily. Picture your orange sacral chakra energy vibrating and clearing as you chant VAAM.

You may begin to feel a stronger libido and desire to be with others as you work with this mantra regularly.

The Solar Plexus Chakra: RAAM (rahm)

The mantra of the solar plexus chakra helps you to cleanse and purify the space of your personal power and ambition. You will be able to have better self-control, avoid negative urges and impulses, bear a confident outlook, and enjoy a balanced level of self-esteem when you chant this mantra.

Picture the bright, yellow light of this energy center getting bigger and warmer, like a sun glowing from within you. By chanting this mantra, or bringing it into your consciousness, you will be increasing your self-esteem right at that moment.

The Heart Chakra: YAAM (yahm)

This mantra for the heart chakra will help you to receive and give love affectively by purifying the energy of the heart. This can have a powerful impact on both physical and spiritual qualities of the heart chakra, eliciting more compassion, unconditional love, and love for the self.

When you chant or intone YAAM, see the bright, green light of this energy center getting bigger and bigger. Picture any blocks floating away from you. (You can also imagine a pink hue if that is your preference)

The Throat Chakra: HAAM (hahm)

The mantra for the throat chakra relieves the impurities and blockages that prevent clear communication and speaking through your true voice. When you can speak clearly from your throat chakra then you can communicate to yourself, as well as the Universe, what you want.

There is also a lot of creativity in this energy field and so you will find that when you can open this chakra and intone HAAM, you will be opening blocks in your creativity as well. Picture the blue light of this chakra releasing any blocks as you connect to this simple mantra.

The Brow (Third Eye) Chakra: AUM/OM (aum/ ohm)

The mantra for the third eye connects to the healing of this energy center and the mind in general. OM is used for a variety of clearing and cleansing needs, and the third eye is an energy center greatly affected by this mantra. The AUM is a similar mantra with a slightly different sound. Both will work well to open you to your inner wisdom, allowing you to be guided by your intuition and follow your true purpose.

Another variation of the third eye chakra is KSHAAM (kah-shahm), which is a mantra for insight and inspiration that will also work well for purifying and balancing your third eye. See the indigo light in the center of your forehead free of any darkness or negativity as you chant any of these mantras to yourself.

The Crown Chakra: OM/AH (ohm/ ahh)

These mantras are both useful for connecting you to the divine and helping heal and cleanse any blocks you may have that stand in the way of that connection. Using these mantras to clear and balance this energy will relieve any feelings of futility, insignificance, and attachment to material things, people, or places.

Several people have suggested that silently intoning this mantra is more effective and you can decide for yourself in your mantra practice. OM will connect you to the divine and AH will help you let go of anything that is being held onto that no longer serves your true purpose and enlightenment.

These seven mantras will help you take a specific focus with each chakra and help heal and rebalance the individual energy centers. There are also mantras that can be used for a general purification and rebalancing and they are:

OM (ohm):

You have already learned about the potential for this mantra to open your third eye and your crown chakras and it is also one of the most universally known mantras that can be applied in a variety of ways. It is considered to be the sound of creation and it affects your energy to help it gather and move in a healthy flow up and outward in the way it needs to go.

OM will help you to open up to and accept your higher-self as it gathers energy and helps you to move that energy upward and outward in a positive flow of life-force.

KRIM (kreem):

This mantra is known to help stimulate the purification, cleansing, and balancing of the lower chakras. This would include the root, sacral, and solar plexus chakras. It can be a good way to start a lower chakra purification and balancing, followed by the individual mantras for each chakra.

SHRIM (shreem):

This mantra connects the most to the head and especially the third eye and crown. It can also be useful as a mantra to elicit feelings of happiness and beauty within the self and the senses.

HRIM (hreem):

This mantra is a powerful tool for opening and awakening the creative self. It widens the capacity for compassion and aids in purifying the heart as well. It can be used in accordance with the sacral and heart chakras separately, or it can be useful for overall balance and meditation.

HUM (hoom):

This mantra will work well to help you dissolve any negative energies and simultaneously helps to promote the flow of positive vibrations, vitality, and positivity throughout the whole body.

All of these mantras can set the tone for your day, your healing journey, and your meditations. You don't have to use all of them at once. In fact, you may need to spend several days or weeks with one or two mantras before trying some of the others, and that is absolutely okay.

In addition to this type of mantra, there are other ways you can invent your own that can be specific to your needs and what you are wanting to heal at the moment. Creating your own mantras will help you connect to your own needs in a powerful way. As a general rule of thumb, keep them simple and try to use less than 10 words when you are making them up. The point is to involve the energy of that mantra in your healing and if it becomes too complicated, your healing process might get complicated too.

Some of the most effective mantras you can use for healing through the chakras are:

I Am Love

To state to yourself in the form of a mantra "I am love" is to become that energy. You are love, the energy of love, and can breathe that energy into everything that you do. This mantra is excellent for opening the heart chakra and the sacral chakra.

I Am Here

In a world full of so many others it can feel overwhelming and sometimes we feel like we are lost in the crowd. We begin to wonder what our purpose is, or if anyone else can see us. The energy of this mantra declares "I am here" so that you can energetically inform your reality that you have the right to take up space. It is particularly useful for opening the solar plexus and the crown chakras.

I Have the Right to See

You have the right to see more than what you are shown. Only you can decide what it is that you want to see and no matter what it is, you have the right to see it. It can be as intense as looking at all of your past lives, or as loving and exciting as seeing yourself in love with another. All of it is your right to look at and identify with on your path of discovery. This mantra is very helpful for awakening and balancing the third eye and the root chakras.

I Have the Right to Ask

Having the right to ask questions also stems from the ability to decide what you want to ask of the world around you. We are all, at one point or another, made to feel like it isn't okay to ask certain questions when in reality it is your right as a citizen of the Universe to ask any question. All of your questions deserve an answer. This mantra helps you resolve any issues you have about questioning the reality of everything and is wonderful for opening up your crown and throat chakras.

We Are All

A simple gesture, the mantra of "We Are All" states that we are all here and we are all everything, and there is no difference between any of us from the perspective of energy. This mantra allows for Universal love, acceptance, and spiritual wisdom. It is the basis of knowing enlightenment and speaks of Universal truth. It is useful for awakening and balancing your crown and heart chakras.

I Trust

This mantra is a bold statement that can be difficult for a lot of people. To trust is to let go of control and give control to the Universe of time, space, and reality. To trust another is to feel totally trusting of yourself as much as you trust another. It is very grounding and results in a new level of freedom. This mantra is effective for clearing and balancing the root and heart chakras.

I Feel

None of us is without emotions and we are often shown by culture and society not to show what we feel too much. It can be very toxic to hold your feelings in and when you are in a balance with yourself you are able to express your emotions in a healthy way. It is part of your human experience to feel and it is your right to do so. The mantra "I Feel" allows you to say to yourself as you are letting go of any other energies that you are capable of feeling and that it is a good thing. This mantra is very empowering to your sacral and heart chakras.

I Am

What more needs to be said? "I am" is incredibly powerful and it says that you are exactly who you need to be right at this moment. You are a presence and you deserve to be here. You are you and that is all you need to be concerned with at this time. The "I am" mantra opens up the channels of all of your chakras as well as the solar plexus, giving bright, sunny yellow light to the power of the self.

Each of these mantras will have an incredibly powerful impact on your energy and as you use them daily or often, you will discover the true way to help heal and balance your chakras. And that's not all you can do. The next chapter will offer a few simple meditations to get you started with some deeper clearing and healing work.

Chapter 12: Meditations for Chakra Balancing and Healing

Within each of your chakras, there are a number of issues and problems that need to be resolved. As you have learned from your reading those imbalances can manifest on the physical, mental, emotional, and spiritual levels. You may already have awareness about which of your chakras are in need of balance and healing and if you are ready to begin your healing process, then this chapter is just for you.

Even if you aren't ready to begin, these meditations will give you an idea of what ways you can begin to align your energies and help yourself feel a lot more energetically positive and light.

For each meditation, you can apply it to the specific chakra you are working with and then the final meditation will be a way for you to align all of the chakras together into one, balanced energy and life-force.

It may be helpful to work with one chakra at a time before attempting to balance the whole system. It will take some daily or regular meditation to get yourself fully healed and that is part of the joy of the journey. The process is an ongoing experience and once you are able to incorporate these tools into regular use, you can keep your chakras healthy, balanced, and whole.

Meditation to Clear Chakras

To begin, find a comfortable place to lie down on the floor. If sitting up is more comfortable for you, that is fine. You can sit cross-legged on the floor or in a chair. If you choose to sit, make sure to keep your spine straight. Otherwise, you can lie on a yoga mat, blanket, or comfortable surface.

Also, make sure you are in a space where you can meditate without disruption. If you need to let people know not to bother you, by all means, tell them. This meditation can be applied to any chakra and so for whichever one you are working on you will picture that energy and work from there.

1. Wherever you have positioned yourself, begin by concentrating on your breath. You will spend several moments connecting to your inhales and exhales. Try doing this for

ten breaths in and ten breaths out at least. Make the breaths deep and long.

2. Now, bring your attention to your body. From the top of your head, down to your toes, release any areas of tension that you are holding onto. Move slowly through each part of the body, an inch at a time. Continue your breathing.

3. When you have come to a full relaxation space, begin to picture all of your chakras from the root to the crown. See the light of each one and ask each of them how they are doing. You don't have to ask out loud; you can simply think the thought.

4. Allow your intuition to pull you in the direction you need to go. It may be that you start at the root, or perhaps at the heart. Wherever you are guided to go is where your intuition is asking you to focus. Lean into that pull.

5. Wherever you are guided, bring your full focus to that chakra and see it as clearly as you can in your third eye (mind's eye). See the color, the light, and see if you can tell if it has any shadows, distortion, or anything else.

6. While you focus on this energy, take a few cycles of inhales and exhales and think about cleansing the energy of the chakra. You can use this opportunity to intone, think, or chant, the mantra for the specific chakra you are in, or you can simply reflect on the energy.

7. You may start to notice certain ideas, thoughts, feelings, and even visual memories or situations pop up as you are meditating on this chakra. This is all good. Don't worry about clearing your thoughts; allow them to come as they are what is rising to the surface to be healed from your energy.

8. Focus on your chakra as these things come up for healing. Whatever rises to your thoughts, feelings, or visions, ask it to be released by picturing it leaving your system and floating through the ceiling or walls, out and away into the Universe.

9. Chant or intone the mantra for this chakra. You can stay in this mantra space as long as you want and when it feels right to stop the mantra, move to the next step.

10. Take several long, deep inhales and exhales. Picture your chakra again and notice if it has changed, or notice if you feel a different energy in yourself.

11. From here, you can either end the meditation or go back to seeing all of your chakras and asking your intuition to guide you to the next space for healing.

*Note: Be careful not to take it too far and overwork your energy. It may be tempting to do all of the chakra meditations in one session; however, this can make healing more challenging. Your energy needs time to adjust after you have worked with a couple of chakras. Be patient and let the healing work have some time to settle after a few days or more, before working with another chakra group.

If you feel guided to work in every chakra, that is between you and your intuition. Just remember that the after-effects of a chakra healing meditation can feel intense. You may feel extra sleepy, exhausted, hungry, emotional, and a variety of other side effects. All of these are normal experiences to have while you are transforming your energy.

Meditation to Bring Balance to Chakras

1. Follow steps 1-4 from the *Meditation to Clear the Chakras*.

2. When you feel pulled to a specific chakra, you will spend time listening to the energy in a similar way that you did before. Close in on that one chakra and look into the light of it with your visualization abilities.

3. Picture the light of the chakra as clear of any shadows or blocks as it rotates in a counter-clockwise direction. This direction is what allows your opening of balance and renewal in this space. The opposing direction, clockwise, is how you will effectively allow your chakras to connect back to each other after the balancing process has occurred.

4. As you imagine the energy flowing in a counter-clockwise direction, like a wheel spinning, all you have to do is breathe for several long, deep inhales and exhales. As your energy swirls, you will be asking the energy of that chakra to reset and renew balance.

5. After you have allowed this rotation for several breaths, begin to shift the direction. It may be too jolting to suddenly switch directions, so use your breath to help the energy to slow and then flow in a clockwise way.

6. Once the energy of the chakra is flowing in a clockwise direction, allow yourself another set of long, deep breaths as you picture the swirling energy.

7. Once you feel a newness in your energy, you can zoom out and picture all of your chakras. You can chant or intone a mantra at this time and close the meditation, or you can ask your intuition to guide you to another chakra for these balancing steps.

8. Spend some time just relaxing on the floor or in your seated position to allow for this energy to incorporate itself into your overall vibration.

Meditation to Align the Chakras as a Whole

For this meditation, you will use all of your assessments with your visualization on the whole system. Rather than picturing one chakra at a time, you will look at the whole system and visualize the healthy flow of energy throughout the entire body, including your auras.

1. Follow steps 1 and 2 in the *Meditation to clear the Chakras.*

2. With your third eye and creative visualization, see all of your chakras from the root to the head, and also picture your entire body.

3. See the chakras in the palms of each hand, on the soles of each foot, and extending above the crown of the head.

4. From there, see your auric field and the light emanating from your body. Can you see any color? What color is your auric field?

5. As you engage with the entire system, continue your deep breathing and picturing the whole body and the colorful light spinning within you and emanating outside of you.

6. See light coming from high in the cosmos, beaming into the crown of the head.

7. Likewise, see light coming up through the earth and beaming into the soles of the feet and palms of the hands.

8. As this light frequency coming from outside of you beams into your energy body, feel it flow through each chakra, one by one, from both the top of the head and the lower extremities.

9. Visualize this light flow circling inside of you, through all of the chakras, like a car on a racetrack. It doesn't have to travel at high speed, the point is to see a closed-loop of energetic current flowing through your whole body, and especially through each chakra.

10. As you continue to inhale and exhale, you will slowly allow the light to slow down and release from your body, allowing the vision

of the light in the crown of your head to return to the cosmos, and the light going through your feet and hands to return to the earth.

11. After you have released that light imagery, spend some time lying, or sitting, and just feel the vibration of light inside of you. Take as long as you want with this sensation.

12. When you are ready to conclude the meditation, you can chant or intone the mantra of 'Om' and then open your eyes.

13. Take your time getting up and drink some water to help your system release more of what your chakras have released in your meditation.

All of these meditations work well for your whole chakra healing journey. They are empowering to your overall energy, as well as the systems that they are responsive to on the physical, mental, emotional and spiritual levels. All you have to do is make time, give space, and breathe through it. Your third eye will do a lot of the hard work for you, so practice your creative visualization skills as this will be one of your greatest tools to help heal your chakras.

In the next chapter, you will learn more about what crystals to use for each chakra and how to incorporate them into your meditation practice.

Chapter 13: Healing Your Chakras with Crystals

The chakras each have their own frequency, as you have learned. Crystals and gemstones also have unique frequencies and there are certain natural correlations between specific chakras and certain crystals. The energy frequency of a balanced chakra will be what you are looking for in the gemstones and crystals you are looking to use in your healing work. That means that the crystals listed in this chapter are radiating the chakra energy you want to balance and shift toward.

The following list is a collection of some of the crystals and gemstones that are specific to each chakra. In your own research, or through other experiences, you may find all kinds of other crystals and stones that will be healing and helpful that may not be listed here. There is a lot to choose from and this is a concise list of where to get you started as you look for the right chakra healing stones for your awakening practice.

Crystals and Gemstones to Balance the Chakras

Crystals and Gemstones for the Root Chakra:

- Bloodstone, Black Kyanite, Fiery Agate, Black Tourmaline, Garnet, Hematite, Obsidian, Smoky Quartz, Tiger's Eye, Red Jasper,

Crystals and Gemstones for the Sacral Chakra:

- Orange Aventurine, Orange Coral, Orange Calcite, Amber, Red Jasper, Carnelian, Snowflake Obsidian, Aragonite, Citrine, Moonstone

Crystals and Gemstones for the Solar Plexus Chakra:

- Yellow Jasper, Amber, Sunstone, Peridot, Lemon Quartz, Citrine, Yellow Tourmaline, Calcite, Quartz Crystal, Malachite, Topaz

Crystals and Gemstones for the Heart Chakra

- Amazonite, Jade, Rose Quartz, Rhodochrosite, Emerald, Green Aventurine, Green Calcite, Green Tourmaline, Rhodonite

Crystals and Gemstones for the Throat Chakra:

- Scolecite, Lapis Lazuli, Celestite Crystal, Blue Calcite, Blue Amazonite, Blue Apatite, Aquamarine, Angelite, Turquoise

Crystals and Gemstones for the for the Brow (Third Eye) Chakra:

- Purple Fluorite, Shungite, Obsidian, Sodalite, Labradorite, Amethyst, Azurite, Quartz Crystal, Black Obsidian

Crystals and Gemstones for the Crown Chakra:

- Diamond, Selenite, White Calcite, Amethyst, Charoite, Kyanite, Quartz Crystal, Sugilite, Lepidolite

So, now that you have an idea of which crystal goes with a chakra, what are you supposed to do with them now? Crystals are a wonderful tool to use in your regular meditations and practices of healing.

You can include any of the crystals you saw from the list into each of your meditations. You can place one stone over the chakra you are planning to focus on or if you are balancing all of them at one time, you can place a stone on each chakra, from the root to the crown.

It is important to allow a nice, relaxing length of time for the crystals and gemstones to do their work. If you are using them with the meditations that you learned from Chapter 12, that length of time will be ample. If you are just going to use them to lie on the floor and clear your mind without doing any visualization work, set a timer for 20-30 minutes of uninterrupted rest with the crystals and gemstones on top of your chakras.

If you want, you can also carry some of them with you as you go out into the world to accomplish your errands, daily tasks, and work. They can be very handy kept in your pocket or somewhere on your person so that the vibration of the crystal is always in contact with your energy throughout the day.

Overall, the energies of crystals are pure and will help you align with the frequencies you are looking for as you work on balancing and healing your energy. Purifying your crystals is something else you can do to keep them in good 'energetic' condition. To purify your stones, you can simply cleanse them in warm salt water for ten minutes, and no more. This is helpful if you use your stones frequently for energy clearing. Many crystals absorb energy and will need purification, too, just as your chakras do.

All of the crystals you see here, and more, will add an extra boost of positive vibration to your chakra healing and awakening. For even more information about the positive effects of chakra healing, the next chapter will give you first-hand knowledge and case studies of people who have begun to thrive again after using these tools and techniques to rebalance their energies and become freer, healthier, and full of joy.

Chapter 14: Case Studies: How Chakra Healing Has Helped So Many

Sometimes we need to see it, to believe it and, in this chapter, I will help you see the truth behind the healing power of chakra awakening through the personal stories of a few of those who have tried these methods and become a happier healthier version of themselves. These case studies are drawn from thousands of people who have healed their suffering by taking their recovery into their own hands by working with their chakras. As you read, you may find similarities to your own experiences or feelings and this section is here to show you that you are not alone in your desire to heal.

Maureen with the Aching World on Her Shoulders

Maureen described her pain as being a discomfort that came from everything that was happening in the world. She watched the news constantly or at least as often as she was able and would feel wrecked by the world of pain, we were all living in. Overtime, Maureen began to have sorrow that led to a level of chronic grief, depression, and anxiety that made it hard for her to feel like her old self.

Her husband asked her to go to a counselor and after a few months she was starting to feel brighter again and then anytime she watched the news, or heard a story about what was happening in the world, she would sink back down into sadness.

Her husband told her not to watch so much of the news and even when she cut herself off, she would still hear about it from her colleagues at the office or her friends at the club.

Finally, Maureen hears about chakra healing and using energy healing methods to help you feel less depressed. At first, Maureen was skeptical and didn't feel confident trying it on her own, so she booked a session with a Reiki practitioner at her local massage parlor. The Reiki practitioner listened to her woes and complaints and explained what energy healing does for a person. After her session, Maureen felt alive and awake in a new way, like she was when she was in her 20's. She was calm and relaxed and feeling positive.

When she heard the news report on her car radio driving home, she heard some awful things and remarked on their sadness to herself, but she did not fall into a deep depression. After her Reiki experience, she decided to try energy healing meditations on her own at home and has been able to maintain a more positive outlook on life ever since.

Tommy and His Insomnia

Tommy suffered from insomnia for the majority of his life. As long as he could remember, he wasn't able to sleep. His parents told him that he was always a good sleeper when he was little, but he doesn't remember that at all. Now in his late 40's, Tommy has adapted to living life without enough sleep. He had to drink large amounts of caffeine to stay awake and functional at his day job and he would often describe himself as a grump because he was always on the edge of tiredness.

Tommy tried all different kinds of sleep aids and medications. He went to a therapist to try and discover the root cause of his insomnia, but never really hit home with it. A friend of his recommended chakra healing therapy and Tommy was reluctant to try anything "too esoteric". His friend sent him a copy of a Chakra Guide he had read to cure his depression and anxiety.

Tommy left it in his email inbox for about 6 months before he finally decided to look. When he began to use the meditations for chakra healing, he had a sudden influx of childhood memories that were hard for him to remember. He began to understand why he had insomnia in the first place and was able to recognize the root cause.

He was afraid of the dark and his father told him that men don't use night lights. He wasn't able to sleep and as a child was given the impression and wound in his chakras that it wasn't okay for him to have what he needed to have a good night's sleep.

That night, Tommy put a night light in his room, just to heal his own childhood wound. He slept for 8 hours straight and woke up a new man. Ever since then, he has discovered more memories to heal through is chakra meditations and no longer suffers from insomnia, nor does he need a night light to sleep.

Carol, Who Thought She'd Never Feel Happy Again

Carol, a mother of 3 and widow to her late husband thought she would never feel happy again. The grief from losing her life partner and being left with their 3 children, a constant reminder of him, was more than she could bear. Carol worked hard to put on a happy face for her kids and when no one was around, she would sob uncontrollably about her husband's passing. After a few years of mourning, her kids getting older and finding more life outside of the house, Carol was left on her own more and the sadness got even worse. She would get lost in memories of when she used to be happy and it would make her feel even sadder.

After seeing a psychiatrist, she was put on antidepressants, as well as a few other prescriptions to help regulate her mood swings and mentality about the loss of her husband. The prescriptions made her lethargic and absent. Her kids were wondering where their mother went.

One of her teenage sons actually talked to her about going to a yoga class with him. She didn't feel up for it, so he offered to teach her at the house. When he got her into and she started trying some of the poses, she began to feel a shift in her energy. She began to smile after he showed her some of the tools for breathing and opening up her chakras. Carol had never heard the word before and got her son to explain it to her.

She began doing research and came across this book, *Chakras Guide*, looking for a way to do more energy healing through her chakras. After using daily meditations and several chakra stones on her own at home, Carol began to feel alive again. She stopped taking prescriptions almost immediately and was able to begin to love her life again, even with her husband gone. She celebrated his life instead of grieving it and found new connections with her kids again.

She continues to practice on herself and even became a Reiki Master to help other people heal from extreme losses as she had experienced in her own life.

Felix Went All the Way

Felix had cancer. Had cancer. He no longer has cancer and here is why. Felix was not interested in chemotherapy. He saw it as a poison that was just as likely to kill him. He chose alternative medicine and methods and began a consistent daily routine with an acupuncturist, a Reiki Master, and a Herbalist.

In addition to visiting these skilled professionals, he used chakra healing crystals, mantras, and meditations, as well as some Yoga and Tai Chi, to connect with his energy and create transformative healing from within.

He was able to recover after about 10 months of daily chakra healing work. His cancer regressed and after an fMRI scan at the end of a year, he was completely cancer-free. He wasn't about to take any chances for cancer to come back, so he kept up his chakra healing practice every day, with his crystals, meditations, bodywork, and other resources.

His life is all about staying in balance on all levels so that he can live cancer-free from now until his age is old. Felix went all the way with chakra healing and awakening, and it healed him all the way.

Conclusion

Thank you for making it through to the end of *Chakras Guide: The Ultimate Beginner's Guide to Chakras and Self-Healing*. Let's hope it was informative and able to provide you with all of the tools you need to achieve your goals whatever they may be. You have traveled on a great journey to discover all of the unique ways your chakras will inform you of what you are in need of and how to change and transform your energy.

The next step is to take this knowledge and apply it to life. You can begin right away and start with the questionnaire from Chapter 7 to help you get a general assessment of your chakra health. If you already have an inkling of where to begin your healing journey, you can jump right to the meditations or go out to your local gem shop and pick up a couple of chakra crystals to empower your healing journey.

The best thing you can do to get started is to try to find a space in every day to listen to your energy and devote as little as 30 minutes clearing your chakra energy. You can create a regular routine, like a morning exercise routine, only for your chakras, and see how you feel after a week or two. I guarantee that if you do a daily chakra clearing meditation every day for two weeks, you are going to notice the difference.

Remember to be patient with your healing journey and give yourself all of the loving care you know you need and deserve as you embrace this great awakening and shift. Your progress depends on you and the energy you put toward healing yourself. If you need outside assistance to keep you in a good balance, find a Reiki practitioner or an acupuncturist in your area, or take a yoga class to help you find some inner peace and chakra healing.

Always remember that as you are healing yourself, support is always available in your community. So many people are using energy healing techniques to empower their transformations and growth through life's ups and downs. You are never alone and all you have to do is say yes! to the healing power of chakra awakening.

Finally, if you found this book useful in any way, a review on Amazon is always appreciated! Good luck on your healing journey!

Copyright © 2019 by Crystal Marcus

www.ingramcontent.com/pod-product-compliance
Lightning Source LLC
Chambersburg PA
CBHW051432250726
48655CB00001B/26